Essentials of Medical Aesthetics and Skin Care

Copyright © 2012 by Dr. Dariush Honardoust. 105822-FERD
Library of Congress Control Number: 2011960643
ISBN: Softcover   978-1-4653-7891-0
            Hardcover   978-1-4653-7892-7

All rights reserved. No part of this book may be reproduced or transmitted in any form or by any means, electronic or mechanical, including photocopying, recording, or by any information storage and retrieval system, without permission in writing from the copyright owner.

To order additional copies of this book, contact:
Xlibris Corporation
1-888-795-4274
www.Xlibris.com
Orders@Xlibris.com

Disclaimer:

Practitioners must always rely on their own experience and knowledge in evaluating and using any information, methods, compounds, or experiments described herein. In using such information or methods they should be mindful of their own safety and the safety of others, including parties, for whom they have a professional responsibility.

With respect to any drug or pharmaceutical products identified, readers are advised to check the most current information provided on procedures featured or by the manufacturers of each product to be administered, to verify the recommended dose or formula, the methods and duration of administration, and contradictions. It is the responsibility of practitioners, relying on their own experience, and knowledge of their patience, to make diagnosis, to determine dosages and the best treatment of each individual patient and to take all appropriate safety precautions.

To the fullest extent of the law, the author shall not assume any liability for any injury and / or damage to persons or property as a matter of products liability, negligence, or otherwise, or from any use or operation of any methods, products, instructions or ideas contained in the material herein.

Essentials of Medical Aesthetics
Clinical and Scientific Skin Care & Rejuvenation

Dr. Dariush Honardoust
Craniofacial/Dental SC, PhD
Faculty of Dentistry, University of British Columbia, Canada
Postdoc, Plastic Surgery Division, University of Alberta, Canada
President of the Canadian Association of Medical Spas and Aesthetic Surgeons

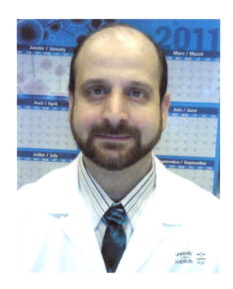

The president and chief director of the Canadian Association of Medical Spas and Aesthetic Surgeons, Dr. Dariush Honardoust, has trained and worked in Canada since 1996. His main interests in the field of aesthetic medicine include nonsurgical face and body contouring, therapeutic and cosmetic botulinum toxin treatment, dermal fillers, chemical peels, and laser cosmetics. His research interests include development of an innovative engineered skin and characterizing the role of small leucine-rich proteoglycans (SLRPs) in the prevention of hypertrophic scar formation after burn, traumatic, acne, and surgical wounds, as well as dermal scars after cosmetic laser operations. Dr. Honardoust has been conducting his research in a wound healing research group and received his doctorate specialty in craniofacial/dental from the Faculty of Dentistry, University of British Colombia, and postdoctoral training from the Department of Reconstructive and Plastic Surgery, University of Alberta, Canada. He is also a consultant-advisor in aesthetic medicine for some Canadian and USA investment firms..

about this text book

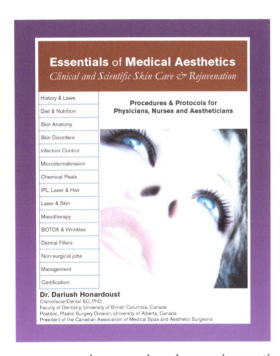

This textbook describes medical aesthetics with discussions of skin anatomy and physiology, methods for the treatment of skin aging and rejuvenation, and the most common skin problems and their management. Each topic gives details further with colored images to assist comprehend and appreciate the details. The book discusses diet and foods associated with skin health, skin types, and the most common skin disorders. In particular, for acne and acne rosacea, etiology, management, and treatment are described. It explains how to differentiate between various types of acne. Those who are interested in scientific information on skin-wound healing can find a comprehensive, yet concise and informative, section in this book. The etiology and types of scar formation after injury are also explained.

The book describes the biology of skin aging (including causes of aging like UV radiation and photoaging) and methods for the improvement of premature skin aging (skin care procedures such as laser rejuvenation, medical chemical peels, and the use of antiaging products). Chemical peels—their types, the grades and different acids used, and their protocols—are discussed broadly to guide how to perform an effective peel. In addition, microdermabrasion and photo-laser and laser hair reduction are thoroughly discussed in this book.

Readers can find complete information on different types of lasers and laser physics. The most appealing areas of medical aesthetics are facial and body countering by derma fillers and Botox injection. This book gives you substantial information about Botox and dermal fillers and the techniques used to perform satisfactory corrective injections. The anatomy and physiology of muscles involved in facial expression are discussed to make you familiar and confident when injecting your clients. For instance, treatment of eyes and forehead wrinkles, frown lines, nasolabial laugh lines, and bunny lines are covered.

The most popular facial and body-countering techniques, such as nonsurgical nose jobs; cheek, chin, and lip enhancements; and nonsurgical breast augmentation and lipolysis by mesotherapy, are presented in this book. The book contains other subjects such as patient consultation and assessment, laser safety, microbiology and medical infection control for medical aesthetics, and other subjects that make this textbook a reference guide in medical aesthetics for doctors, nurses, and aestheticians.

table of contents

Chapters

1.	Introduction to Medical Aesthetics	9
2.	Anatomy and Physiology of Skin	27
3.	Nutrition and Skin Rejuvenation	43
4.	Most Common Skin Problems	55
5.	Microbiology for Medical Aestheticians	95
6	Skin Rejuvenation Procedures	107
7	Laser Cosmetics	127
8.	Facial Muscle Anatomy and Physiology	147
9.	Botulinum Toxin Cosmetic (BOTOX)	155
10.	Dermal Fillers (Injectables)	173

chapter 1

Introduction to Medical Aesthetics

DEFINITION OF THE MEDICAL AESTHETICS

ABOUT THE AESTHETICS MEDICINE

ROLE OF MEDICAL AESTHETICIANS

PROFESSIONAL TEAMWORK

MEDICAL AESTHETICIAN AUTHORITY

AESTHTICIANS AND BUSINESS

MEDICAL AESTHETICS CLIENTS

MEDICAL AESTHETICS CERTIFICATION

WHY CERTIFICATION IS IMPORTANT?

MEDICAL AESTHETICS TRAINING PROGRAM

MEDICAL SPA CLINICS

MEDICAL SPA CLASSIFICATION

PATIENTS' STATEMENT OF RIGHTS

CHOOSING A RIGHT MEDICAL SPA/COSMETIC CLINIC

CLIENTS' RESPONSIBILITIES

PREPARE TO ANSWER CRITICAL QUESTIONS ABOUT YOUR CLINIC

DOS AND DON'TS IN CHOOSING THE RIGHT MED SPA

MEDICAL SPA MANAGEMENT

CHAPTER 1

Introduction to Medical Aesthetics

DEFINITION OF THE MEDICAL AESTHETICS

Since decades ago, Chinese intellectuals originally have been trying to develop basic cosmetology thoughts that extrapolate in medicine. Today, this area of practice is considered as a distinct subdivision of medicine, namely "medical aesthetics." The English term *aesthetic* reflects to the factors concerning or characterized by an appreciation of beauty or good taste. This definition appears primarily as a result of the growing evidence of people who employ beauty and health in harmony with the current knowledge in the relevant medical practice. A main purpose of medical aesthetics is to improve the quality of beauty in conjugation with health and medical procedures and to enhance excellence in both health and beauty.

Figure 1.1

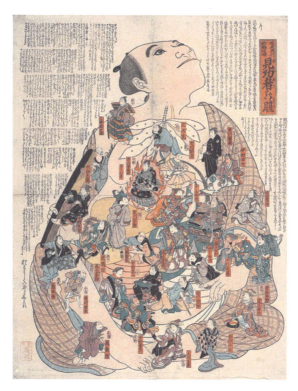

Courtesy of http://pinktentacle.com
Bodily functions and beauty personified as popular kabuki actors (artist unknown, late 19th century)

ABOUT THE AESTHETICS MEDICINE

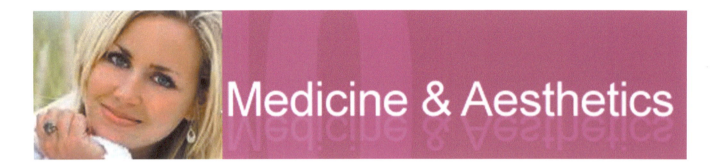

Medical aestheticians possess high-technology skin care that represents the blend of health care and beauty services. They use advanced technologies to provide a medically based procedure designed to implement a noteworthy cosmetic change or enhancement. Services offered by medical aestheticians can involve the use of lasers or other energy-based devices. In other words, medical aestheticians are practitioners in cosmetology that specialize in scientific skin care and rejuvenation. Care of the body's largest organ, skin, has spanned from ancient days to highly technological, up-to-date science administered by cosmetic and plastic surgeons and professional medical aestheticians. Therefore, a medical aesthetician needs an extensive knowledge based on current scientific skin types, physiology, and pathology.

A medical aesthetician must also understand contraindications, product usage, the diversity of techniques and equipment to be used in the treatment, skills, and expertise in order to recommend the best treatments to the client. It encompasses knowledge of skillful massage techniques to help improve skin functions as well as providing a relaxing experience for the client. Over the past recent years, the medical aesthetic industry continues to see a remarkable quantity of expansion. This exponential growth has led to a very high demand for medical aestheticians to work at medical spas or cosmetic medicine centers.

A medical aesthetician works along with medical doctors or registered nurses. The responsibilities rotate around treating patients with both medical conditions and cosmetic needs. Under supervision, a medical aesthetician can utilize medical-grade devices as well as products. A medical aesthetician may also assist the cosmetic physicians or dermatologists for injectables and nonsurgical facial enhancement. Due to the constant growth of this industry, the demand for medical aestheticians is escalating. Therefore, obtaining medical training is required for salon and spa technicians to make them qualified for being a medical aesthetician. Very often, medical directors in the facilities train the aesthetician either during the employment or prior to starting in order to bring the aesthetician up to speed on the medical procedures and terminology. However, it is required to seek training in one of the recognized medical aesthetics institutes before working as a formal medical aesthetician.

ROLE OF MEDICAL AESTHETICIANS

Over the decades, physicians and their colleagues have developed a wide range of procedures to help reduce the manifestation of wrinkles and the undesirable effects associated with skin aging. The fame of facial rejuvenation is indisputably accountable for a new generation of health care practitioners who supplement the plastic surgeon's skill in serving clients who seek aesthetic treatment. Medical aestheticians have become valuable assets within medical spas or aesthetic clinics. In addition to supporting the goals of surgeons, they play a role as advocates for patients and work to accomplish the best possible surgical outcomes for clients.

Figure 1.2

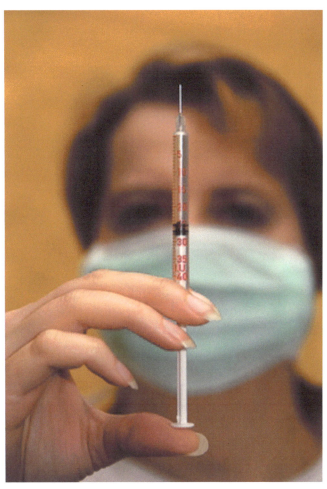

Medical aestheticians are skin care technicians who work in the spa industry or along with physicians offering treatments such as facials and chemical peels. Physicians often seek to hire nurses trained as aestheticians to offer laser treatments and cosmetic injections in their practice. Nurses who have an interest in helping clients improve their physical appearance seek training to transition into this career..

PROFESSIONAL TEAMWORK

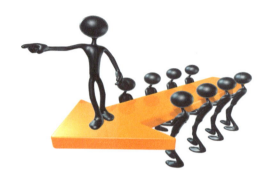

Professional support has become an essential part before and after the performance of aesthetic procedures to help prepare the patient for surgery, enhance the healing process, and ensure a more contented client. Medical aestheticians progress beyond the typical territory of skin care to assist the surgeon in different treatment settings such as medical spas, surgery clinics, and hospitals. Enhanced service, which leads to greater client satisfaction, is one of the most important benefits of integrating a medical aesthetician into the cosmetic surgery practice.

Excellence of service and safety are key fundamentals for people who seek out facial rejuvenation. It has been proven that if problems arise after the surgery, the clients are less likely to take legal actions if they have received consistent support and attention from the commencement of the process. Prior to surgery, the medical aesthetician can provide support to clients who become apprehensive in anticipation of the procedures results. The aesthetician can also educate the client how to proceed for skin care before and after surgery in order to optimize the healing process.

MEDICAL AESTHETICIAN AUTHORITY

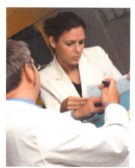

Medical aestheticians must provide informational support for both the surgeon and the client. Educating the patient before surgery is critical. The medical aesthetician must function as the expert and specialized skin care practitioner within the medical spa or surgery clinic facility to not only provide traditional medical support but also offer services such as clinical skin treatment pre- and postoperation, progressive supervision, postsurgical makeup to increase the client comfort level, and dietary direction. The medical aesthetician must be systematically familiar with the patient's skin type and record. The highlights of medical aestheticians skills should include laser facial treatments, chemical peeling, microdermabrasion, and general aesthetic and reconstructive procedures.

AESTHTICIANS AND BUSINESS

Employing a professional medical aesthetician in the practice is a thoughtful business decision that can contribute to consistent long-term income. The increase in income can include both skin treatments and skin care–product sales, leading to greater profitability. Therefore, a medical aesthetician whose personality can positively influence the clients is one of the most important assets in of a medical spa.

The aesthetician, however, must appreciate the medical spa commerce and be capable of assist other personnel in the office, if needed. To help attain the long-term goals for the practice, the clinic owner and/or employer should keep the aesthetician up to date about new techniques in skin rejuvenation procedures. The aesthetician can, in turn, teach patients about new procedures and products.

MEDICAL AESTHETICS CLIENTS

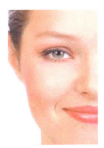

As the baby boomer generation reaches their fifties, the demand for antiaging services has increased significantly. The ability to provide striking benefits without surgery has been a perfect match for this part of the society. The resulting rise in the number of medical spas or medical aestheticians has made these procedures easily accessible and increases their popularity. Most importantly, since these enhancements can be made without anesthesia, downtime, or significant discomfort, the number of clients who desire to undergo the procedures is escalating.

Americans spent over $12 billion on cosmetic procedures last year. The ASAPS (American Society for Aesthetic Plastic Surgery) reported 10.2 million cosmetic procedures in 2009. Since the Aesthetic Society started collecting multispecialty procedural statistics in 1997, they reported the overall number of cosmetic procedures has increased 162%. The most frequently performed nonsurgical procedure was Botox injections, and the most popular surgical procedure was breast augmentation. Top nonsurgical cosmetic procedures among men and women in 2009 were as follows:

- botulinum toxin: 2,464,123
- laser hair removal: 1,280,964
- dermal filler: 1,262,848
- chemical peel: 591,808
- laser skin resurfacing: 570,880

MEDICAL AESTHETICS CERTIFICATION

Certification is a method to elevate the status and legitimacy among peers and other medical personnel and demonstrate competency with potential and existing government regulatory agencies. For physicians, board certification may be necessary to gain or maintain privileges in performing medical aesthetic surgery at a particular firm, to demonstrate a level of competency greater than others in the field, and to demonstrate that practitioners are interested in setting and maintaining high standards of client care. For medical aestheticians, certification may be necessary as well because clinics or physicians may require certification for employment. In addition, medical aestheticians can demonstrate a level of competency equal to or greater than others in the field through certification.

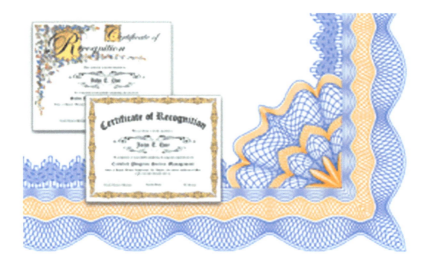

WHY CERTIFICATION IS IMPORTANT?

Certification is an affirmation that one has completed a course of study, passed an examination, or otherwise met specified criteria for certification. However, certification is not permission to act but, rather, a statement of completion or qualification. Certification is a private matter, issued by a private organization that provides the clients with more information and confidence about the certified practitioner. It also gives practitioners a way to increase their competency through passing a course of study and exams and for advertising or informing their colleagues and the public of their qualification of performance in the certified subject.

MEDICAL AESTHETICS TRAINING PROGRAM

With the prompt advances in the field of skin care and medical cosmetic procedures, the critical need for both education and special certification is substantially increasing. A standard medical aesthetics training program should provide both basic core information and advanced practical knowledge in medical aesthetics. The program must offer potentials of employment and professional occupation for makeup artists, holistic health practitioners, cosmetologists, nurses, aestheticians, medical or lab assistants, and medical doctors who wish to extend their business beyond their general practice.

Thus, a medical aesthetics certification program should be able to train medical doctors and registered nurses who wish to expand their qualifications in the areas of aesthetic medicine and to practice nonsurgical/noninvasive procedures in medical spa clinics. Other medical or paramedical educators may attend the program and obtain the certification of completion; however, in most circumstances they must work under the supervision of qualified physicians, board-certified surgeons, or licensed dermatologists when working close to the areas of injectables and/or botulinum toxin.

Table 1.1: A summary of the core courses that should be included in a medical aesthetics training program

Core courses in a standard medical aesthetics training program
Anatomy and Physiology for the Aestheticians
Skin, Nails, and Hair Disorders
Client Assessment for Medical Aesthetics
Microbiology and Sanitization
Cosmetic Lasers and Physics (Laser Hair Removal; Laser Tattoo Removal)
Chemical Peels
Dermal Fillers
Cosmetic and Therapeutic Botox
Microdermabrasion and Laser Skin Resurfacing
Skin Care Products and Chemistry
Medical Spa Safety and Regulations
Practice and Hands-On Training
Medical Spa Business and Management

MEDICAL SPA CLINICS

Due to the growth of the aesthetic medical procedures' popularity over the past several years, such procedures are increasingly being performed in nonclinical environments such as offices in shopping malls, beauty salons, or day spas. It is recognized that combining cosmetics with medical procedures may be acceptable for enhancing the business and provides an additional level of handiness and expediency to patients. However, a regulatory structure is desirable to ensure proper medical practice and clientele protection. As a general standard for the health care professional that performs the procedures, the proposed regulations presented here review the guidelines developed, recognized, and employed by worldwide health care professional organizations.

Figure 1.3

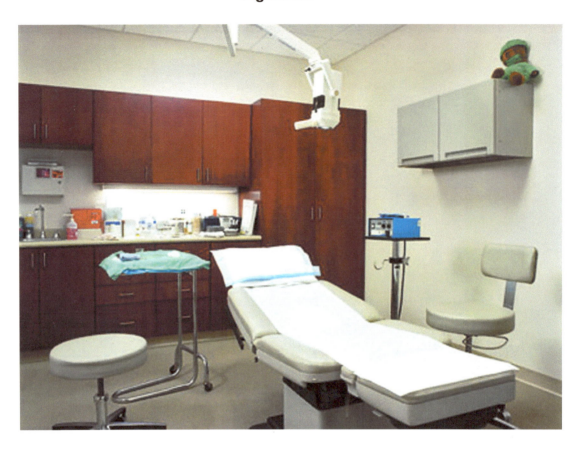

A medical spa clinic should provide high level of service and safety, showcase a broad range of advanced diagnostics and therapeutics available, enhance patient education and awareness, and demonstrate compliance with the highest governing operational standards of professional excellence.

MEDICAL SPA CLASSIFICATION

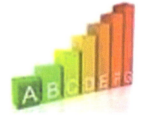

Echelon I Medical Spas

Echelon I medical spas include those facilities in which only superficial procedures are performed. The procedures affect only the uppermost layer of skin, with no invasive methods. It is recommended that all personnel be certified in basic cardiac life support. The Basic Life Support for Healthcare Providers addresses core material such as adult and pediatric CPR; foreign-body airway obstruction; automated external defibrillator (AED) use; and stroke, cardiac arrest, and special resuscitation situations.

Echelon II Medical Spas

Echelon II includes those medical spas in which procedures with a higher risk of unfavorable consequences are performed, including Botox and dermal-filler injections and use of lasers. However, the risk of hospitalization due to these procedures is unlikely. Echelon II spas must maintain basic emergency equipment and procedures. All personnel must be certified in basic cardiac life support and at least one health care professional who has completed a course in advanced cardiac life support must be present in the clinic at all times. The purpose of ACLS is to prepare health care providers for initiating advanced resuscitative efforts in response to cardiovascular emergencies experienced by adults. At the end of the ACLS program, the successful learner will have demonstrated both the required knowledge and skills to manage cardiorespiratory emergencies using the systematic ACLS approach.

Echelon III Medical Spas

Echelon III medical spas include those facilities in which procedures may have complications of a serious nature and may permanently alter the skin or underlying tissue, remove tissue, and/or involve injection or use of devices and products that require specific and high levels of professional training. A licensed physician must be on the premises and available to respond at all times. All personnel must be certified in basic cardiac life support, and at least one health care professional who has completed a course in advanced cardiac life support must be present in the clinic at all times.

PATIENTS' STATEMENT OF RIGHTS

Medical spa staff should recognize the basic rights of patients and value patients' rights. A patients' rights document should be available upon request. The following rights are intended to serve the patient, his or her family, and/or representatives or legal guardian(s). These rights must be promoted and protected by both clients and clinical staff:

1. High-quality care delivered in a safe and efficient manner.
2. Treatment in accordance with accepted standards of courtesy.
3. Respect of privacy and confidentiality.
4. Information on diagnosis, treatment options, and prognosis.
5. The risks, benefits, and possible complications of each treatment or procedure.
6. Information on the qualifications of those who will be performing the procedures.
7. The right to refuse treatment and advice on the consequences of this decision.
8. Inspection and obtainment of a copy of medical records and the billing.
9. Requesting information regarding alternative appropriate care.
10. Knowing the expectations of manners and the consequences of not complying with these expectations.

CHOOSING A RIGHT MEDICAL SPA/COSMETIC CLINIC

A medical spa is a cross between a doctor's office and a day spa, with all procedures carried out under the supervision and authority of a licensed medical doctor. However, not all medical spas provide same quality service and care to the clients. Visiting a med spa should be fun, relaxing, and productive and not result in a visit to the emergency room, infection, or permanent scarring. While the noninvasive treatments carried out at most med spas have less risk of complication than full-on plastic or cosmetic surgery, serious injury could still occur.

Figure 1.4

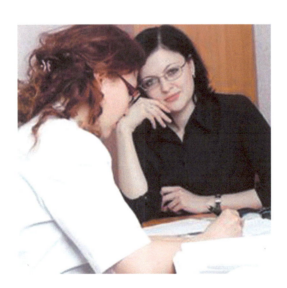

Patient's rights outline the rights of any patient receiving medical care, including surgical or nonsurgical cosmetic procedures. The laws protect the rights of clients in a medical aesthetics facility and require the facility to provide the patient with a copy of these rights prior to treatment if requested.

CLIENTS' RESPONSIBILITIES

In a discussion of patients' rights, it's also important to review patients' responsibilities. Medical aesthetics clients have the right to choose their means for paying for their treatments, and that right is balanced by the responsibility of taking care of those payments or corresponding financial obligations. There is no question that aesthetics costs can become difficult and cumbersome, but they do need to be dealt with responsibly. Candidates for cosmetic procedures should recognize that being totally honest with practitioners is imperative. This means sharing all information about habits and health as holding back can mean not getting the care that they need. Below outlines the responsibilities of patients who are considering undergoing the desired procedures:

1. Provide a complete health history
2. Participate in treatment and services
3. Communicate with staff
4. Comply with doctor's or doctors' treatment plan
5. Be courteous to other clients and staff
6. Accept the treating room assignments
7. Accept physician, nurse, clinician, and other caregiver assignments
8. Protect belongings
9. Arrange for transportation home
10. Make payments for services
11. Keep your appointments

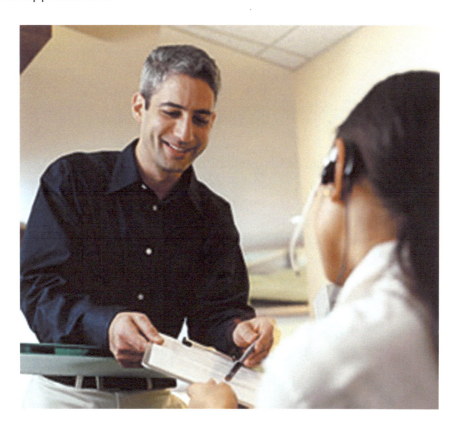

PREPARE TO ANSWER CRITICAL QUESTIONS ABOUT YOUR CLINIC

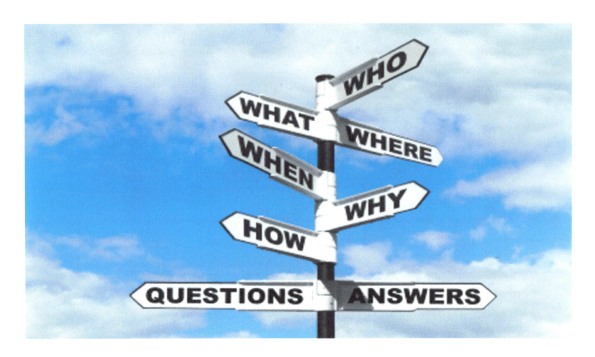

Is a doctor available in the medical spa?

Medical treatments must be carried out only with full medical supervision. However, often the doctor is not on-site. Unlicensed personnel with a basic training in a specific procedure should not work on the clients. A licensed full-time medical director and nurse on-site, preferably in the room with clients or at least in a supervisory position overseeing qualified medical personnel, must be present in the facility. The author recommends that the doctor be a licensed family physician, a dermatologist, a qualified dentist, or a plastic surgeon.

Is the staff experienced in specific procedures?

A medical spa may have several years of experience overall but only a short period of time experience in the procedure a specific client wants to have carried out. They want to find out who their practitioner will be; how many times he or she has carried out the specific procedure they want in the last year, month, and week; how often serious side effects occur; check credentials; and finally ask about training and background. Professional and caring staff should not feel insulted by the questions.

Is the consultation up to standard?

Medical spas usually must encourage their patients to ask as many questions as they need to until they feel entirely comfortable and give them up-to-date information. Consultations should be one-on-one with a medical professional and should leave clients feeling satisfied with the outcome.

What is the equipment like?

The equipment should be up-to-date, well-maintained, sterile, and the right choice available for different skin types. The equipment should be clean, and the entire facility should be hygienic, with proper hand-sterilizing facilities available for both clients and personnel.

Are clients satisfied overall?

If clients return for repeat visits because they are satisfied with the medical spa's reputation and practice, it is a good sign to rely on. If they are interested in one specific procedure, they may ask if the medical spa can provide contact details of satisfied patients. A confident doctor would not mind doing this.

Is the price right?

Medical spas that make impossible promises or offer prices that are significantly cheaper than other places in the same area will be questioned more on details to make sure that they provide a standard and acceptable level of service. Medical spa personnel who want to sell a series of treatments are often asked to give the clients more freedom and comfort levels to decide given the budget that they have set aside for their cosmetics needs.

DOS AND DON'TS IN CHOOSING THE RIGHT MED SPA

1. Do take your time in finding a medical spa that is right for you, makes you feel comfortable, and where the staff is fully trained, certified, and licensed.
2. Don't go for the lowest-price option. If a price is way too low, you have the right to become suspicious and investigate more, considering that the procedure is going to be performed on your body and it is not just buying a new dress or fancy pair of shoes.
3. Do make sure the clinic or facility in question is devoted to medical spa procedures and aesthetics in general.
4. Do make sure that all medical procedures are performed by medical personnel, not unlicensed or nonmedical staff. Check laws to see if procedures such as giving injections and doing deep chemical peels must be performed by a doctor, or if nursing staff can carry them out under a doctor's supervision. And if you see an untrained secretary giving injections or doing a chemical peel, don't be afraid to report them.
5. Don't go to someone's home, a hotel room, or a temporary rented space for a medically related treatment. The Canadian Association of Medical Spas and Aesthetic Surgeons recommends only visiting a med spa located within a physician's office.

MEDICAL SPA MANAGEMENT

Medical Spa Marketing

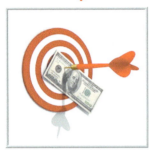

Besides clinical skills, one of the most important aspects of being successful as medical aestheticians is advanced training that focuses on attracting and maintaining clients. As recent business in the aesthetics field become increasingly more competitive, medical aestheticians need to focus on innovative ideas to increase their contribution to the business. This information is just as essential for beginners in the field as it is for the experienced experts. Due to practical awareness and technical improvements, the delivery of medical procedures and services is faster and less invasive than before. This is especially true in the area of minimally invasive cosmetic procedures that use botulinum toxin and dermal-filler injections, microdermabrasion, and intense pulsed light (IPL) to provide skin care services.

One of the client-friendly approaches in aesthetic medicine is in offering follow-up visitations and outpatient treatment services to meet the practical needs of the clients, whose view of health has developed to include more than traditional medicine offers. Many view beauty and health as harmonizing areas that generate a new sense of wellness. Therefore, medical cosmetic clients expect more accomplishments than just solving a health-related problem. It should provide a feeling of overall well-being. The medical spa industry is dedicated to delivering a medical practice in a spa setting. The quality management of the business relationships of these types of centers is all about creating organized services in a reputable medical practice.

Legal Affairs and Liabilities

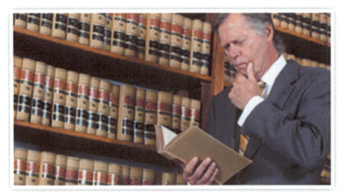

New technologies have brought smaller and more affordable equipment that require less space and reduced funds. However, medical spa owners need to be aware of several legal and regulatory issues that involve safety, security, and permission for using such equipment and products at all levels of government. Each treatment in the practice has to be approved by an appropriate governing organization. However, regulations for the administration of these types of procedures vary widely from county to county. Although a responsible medical director should be familiar with these laws, all members of management should be aware of the specific regulations for the region in which they practice.

Focusing on the Clients

The medical spa owner has to identify the business's core clientele based on the demographics of the surrounding area and then must design its marketing and business operations around that type of client. The focus may not be on maximizing the number of appointments booked but on providing fewer clients with longer, more relaxing experiences yet faster procedures. The spa's owner, manager, and medical director must synchronize their endeavors in order to stabilize the direction of the facility. The occurrence of negligence on any medical practice may result in serious legal consequences that hinder the medical spa from its normal operations. To avoid this, the management team must assure that the medical personnel have individual malpractice insurance plans of their own. However, this will not protect the spa itself, which needs to secure its own separate coverage.

Management Responsibility

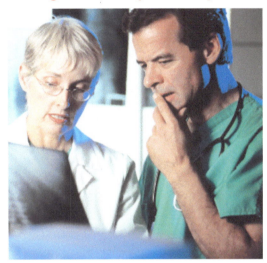

Specific essentials of the affiliation between the spa manager and the medical director must be established before commencing a medical spa business. In the majority of cases, the medical director must supervise all aspects of the medical practice in an independent manner, establish high-quality standards for governing medical procedures, and train the staff accordingly. In the meantime, the facility manager should focus on conducting business operations and on creating a customer service–oriented environment. This can include engaging and educating the nonmedical employees to ensure that they indulge clients and make them feel comfortable before, during, and after the procedures.

In addition, the spa manager has to coordinate practices that discriminate the business from a traditional physician's office. It is well desired that clients be able to make appointments within a week, and follow-up visits should be scheduled conveniently. Wait times for those appointments should be minimized considerably from those that are experienced at typical medical offices. Some of the duties of a nonmedical manager of a medical spa include day-to-day business operations, such as bookkeeping, ordering nonmedical supplies, and dealing with landlord and space issues. However, the two parties must balance the reputation versus the cost of the equipment used in the facility

Client Satisfaction

Meeting the needs of the spa's core clientele is essential. Here are some important tips that will enhance the client satisfaction:

- *Recording* of the types of people receiving treatments
- *Monitoring* core clients changing from your initial target segment
- *Offering* loyalty programs, including referral discounts, frequent customer rewards, and rebates
- *Attracting* new customers by investments of time and funds in marketing, promotions, and general relationships
- *Conducting* local events at which the spa can demonstrate its services
- *Presenting* its own event to draw clients
- *Exploring* other partnerships with related services, such as laser eye surgery and cosmetic dentistry

Figure 1.5

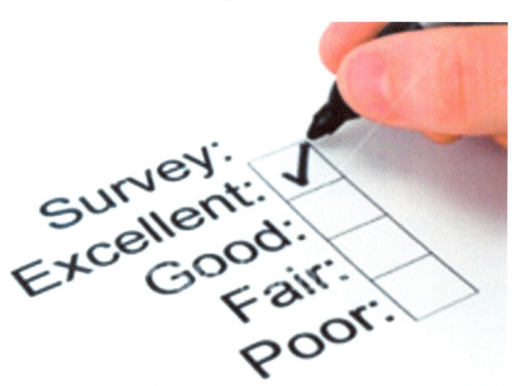

Clients' satisfaction is important for a medical spa to maintain its customer flow and compete with other centers.

chapter 2

Anatomy and Physiology of Skin

HUMAN SKIN

EPIDERMIS

DERMIS

HYPODERMIS

EPIDERMAL APPENDAGES

HAIR FOLLICLES

SEBACEOUS GLANDS

SWEAT GLANDS

SKIN-WOUND HEALING

HEMOSTASIS

INFLAMMATORY RESPONSE

REEPITHELIALIZATION

GRANULATION TISSUE

SKIN-TISSUE REMODELLING

HAIR-GROWTH CYCLE

HAIR DISORDERS

HAIR LOSS (ALOPECIA)

EXCESSIVE HAIRINESS (HIRSUTISM)

MELANOCYTES AND SKIN COLOR

NAILS

CHAPTER 2

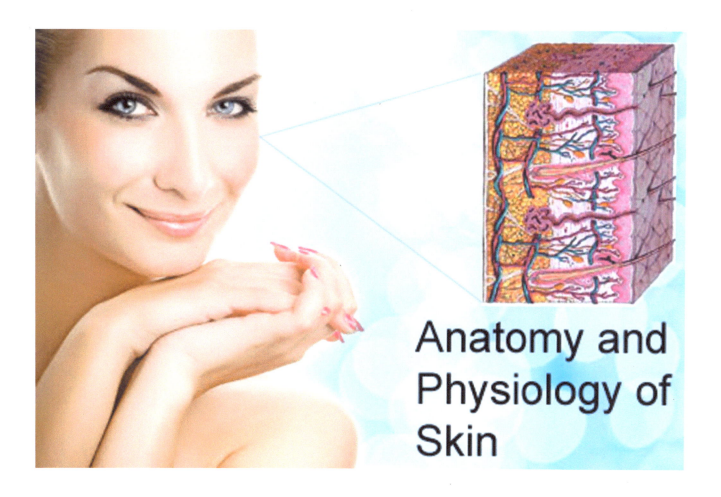

Anatomy and Physiology of Skin

HUMAN SKIN

Human skin is the largest organ and covers the entire outside of the body. An adult's skin weighs roughly six pounds. In addition to providing a protective shield against physical and environmental factors such as heat, light, injury, and microorganisms, the skin also regulates body temperature; stores water, fat, and vitamin D; and serves as a delicate comprehension sensor for pain and pleasant stimulations. Throughout the body, the skin's physical characteristics vary in terms of thickness, color, and texture. For example, the head contains more hair follicles than anywhere else while the soles of the feet contain none. However, the soles of the feet and the palms of the hands have greater thickness. The skin is made up of three distinct layers: epidermis, dermis, and hypodermis.

EPIDERMIS

The epidermis is a stratified squamous epithelium and the most outer layer of the skin that consists primarily of cells called keratinocytes. The epidermis is comprised of five sublayers, which from top to bottom are named the stratum corneum, the stratum lucidum, the stratum granulosum, the stratum spinosum, and the stratum basale (Figure 2.1). The stratum corneum is made of dead flat keratinocytes that shed continuously about every two weeks. The stratum basale of the basal layer is the inner layer of the epidermis that contains basal germinative cells. They continually divide and push already formed cells into higher layers and, hence, replaces the old ones that are shed from the top layer. As the cells move into the higher layers, they grow, differentiate, flatten, and eventually die. No blood vessels exist in the epidermis, and the underlying dermis provides nutrients and removes metabolic waste by diffusion through the cell junctions.

DERMIS

The dermis is the middle layer of the skin. Compared to the epidermis, the dermis has a more complex structure and is composed of two layers: the superficial papillary dermis and the deep reticular dermis (Figure 2.2). The dermis acts as a base to maintain and hold the epidermis. The papillary dermis is thinner and consists of loose connective tissue capillaries, collagen, and elastic fibers. The connective tissue of the reticular dermis is thicker and denser and contains larger blood vessels and coarse collagen bundles fibers that are arranged parallel to the surface. The dermis also contains fibroblasts, mast cells, nerve endings, lymphatics, and epidermal appendages.

The blood vessels transport blood, which supplies important nutrients to the skin, and the nerves allow perception of sensations like pain, temperature, and touch. Fibroblasts are the major cell types that synthesize collagen and other extracellular matrix molecules. The substance background of the dermis is composed of hyaluronic acid, glycoproteins, and chondroitin sulfate glycosaminoglycans. The deep surface of the dermis is highly irregular and borders the adipose tissue or fat subcutaneous layer.

HYPODERMIS

The hypodermis is the lowermost layer of skin tissue and is also known as the subcutaneous layer. Major cell types found in the hypodermis are fibroblasts, adipose cells, and macrophages. The hypodermis is used mainly for fat storage. The structure of the hypodermis is comprised of a network of collagen and adipose cells that conserve the body's heat while protecting other organs from injury by acting as a shock absorber. Thus, this fat layer assists in the course of homeostasis by forming a layer of insulation to sluggish heat loss.

Figure 2.1: Structure of epidermis

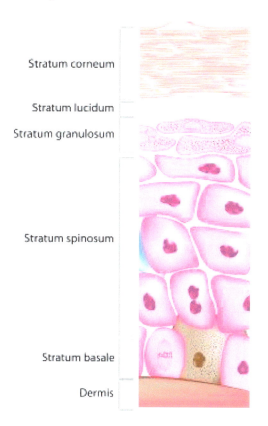

The stratum corneum is the outermost of the five layers of the epidermis and is largely responsible for the vital barrier function of the skin. It is the key to healthy skin and its associated attractive appearance. Keratinocytes arise in the deepest level of the epidermis, and new cells are constantly being produced. As this happens, the older cells migrate up to the surface of the skin and are eventually worn off.

Figure 2.2: Layers of the skin

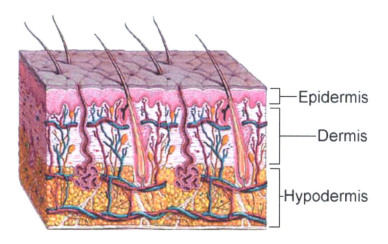

Three layers of the skin are epidermis, dermis, and hypodermis. The epidermis is the skin's primary defense against the environment. The dermis is primarily composed of collagen and elastin fibers, which provide the skin with structure, support, and elasticity. Hypodermis or subcutaneous tissue is composed of fat (adipose tissue).

EPIDERMAL APPENDAGES

Epidermal appendages include hair follicles, sweat glands, sebaceous glands, apocrine glands, and mammary glands. They often can be found in the deep dermis and provide cells that differentiate for the generation of the new epidermis. Remarkably, these epidermal appendages may be found in the subcutaneous fat beneath the dermis in the face. Thus, even in deep dermal wounds of the face, reepithelialization occurs to promote the healing process.

HAIR FOLLICLES

Hair follicles are complex structures formed by the epidermis and dermis. They can be found over the entire area of the skin with some exceptions. The structure of a hair follicle consists of the papilla, the matrix, the root, the sheath, and the hair fiber. The papilla is mainly made up of connective tissue and a capillary ring at the base of the follicle. Melanocytes and epithelial cells comprising the hair matrix surround the papilla. Melanocytes are responsible for skin and hair color mediated by the pigment melanin. Two types of human hair melanin are eumelanin in black or brown hair and pheomelanin in blond hair. Hair fiber cells and the inner root sheath are originated from the hair matrix.

These cells are the fastest growing cell populations in the human body. Hair matrix cells continually multiply upward, dehydrate, and are packed into a dead dense, hard matter that forms the hair shaft. Chemotherapy and/or radiotherapy often lead to the death of hair matrix dividing cells and temporary hair loss. A fragile covering, namely the cuticle, is composed of plate-like scales covering the hair shaft. The hair fiber consists of an intermediate cortex and an inner medulla. Other structures associated with the hair follicle include arrector pili muscles. The sympathetic nervous system controls the contraction of arrector pili muscles, leading to the vertical orientation of the follicle and the hairs to stand. The hair follicle also senses the position of the hairs by its receptors.

Figure 2.3: Anatomy of a hair follicle

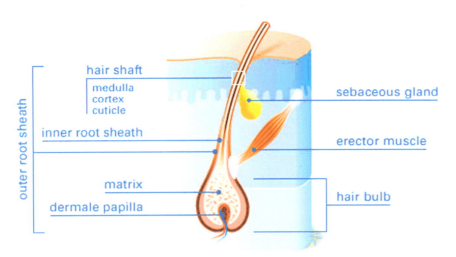

The matrix contains rapidly dividing keratinocytes, which give rise to the keratinized hair shaft. The hair follicle melanocytes reside in the lower part of the hair bulb among the matrix keratinocytes. The matrix is in the deepest portion of the follicle, which envelops the dermal papilla. The bulge area is comprised of follicle stem cells. Melanocytes transfer packets of melanin to the hair follicle matrix keratinocytes, which confers color to the hair shaft.

Asian people have vertically oriented follicles that produce straight hairs whereas the hair follicles of black-skinned individuals are oriented parallel to the skin surface. Caucasian hair follicles are oriented at an angle to the skin surface. Finally, the bulge located in the outer root sheath at the insertion point of the arrector pili muscle encompasses a number of stem cell types that provide the entire hair follicle with new cells and are involved in reepithelialization during wound healing.

SEBACEOUS GLANDS

Sebaceous glands can be found in the entire surface of the skin except the palms, the soles, and the dorsum of the feet. By contrast, they are largest and most concentrated in the facial skin, the scalp, and at the sites of acne. Sebaceous glands secrete skin oils, including triglycerides, fatty acid breakdown products, wax esters, squalene, cholesterol esters, and cholesterol. These oily substances lubricate the skin to protect against abrasion and roughness, hence making it more resistant to moisture.

SWEAT GLANDS

Figure 2.4: Structure of a sweat gland

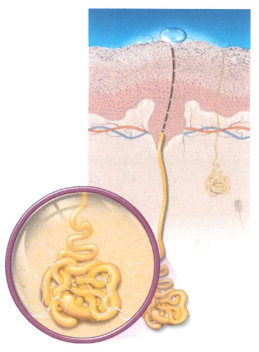

Sweat glands can be found over the entire surface of the skin except at the vermillion border of the lips, the external ear canal, the nail beds, and the glans of the penis. Sweat glands are most concentrated in palm soles and armpits. Each gland is comprised of a looped secretory part that links to the epidermis through a distal duct. Upon stimulation of the thermoregulatory center in the hypothalamus when temperature reaches or exceeds a set point, the sweat glands are activated through sympathetic nerve fibers that innervate the sweat glands, resulting in the production of sweat.

Sweating lowers the body temperature through the absorption of the heat from the surface of the body while it evaporates. Sweat glands are divided into two types: apocrine and eccrine. Apocrine glands can be found over the entire body, whereas eccrine glands can be found most commonly in the underarms, the breasts, and the area between the thighs and abdomen.

Each gland consists of a tiny tube that originates as a ball-shaped coil in the dermis or in the subcutaneous layer of the skin. The coiled portion of the gland is closed at its deep end and is lined with sweat-producing cells.

SKIN-WOUND HEALING

The process of wound healing is comprised of overlapping phases of inflammation and repair in which platelets, fibroblasts, epithelial cells, endothelial cells, and inflammatory cells interact with each other and extracellular matrix (ECM) molecules, growth factors, and cytokines. Aberrations in this process may result in chronic nonhealing wounds or deposition of excess collagen and scar formation. Wound healing consists of three partially overlapping phases: (a) hemostasis and inflammation, (b) reepithelialization and granulation tissue formation, and (c) maturation and tissue remodeling. Figure 2.7 summarizes major wound-healing events over time.

HEMOSTASIS

Soon after wounding, glycoproteins expressed on the cell surface of platelets mediate their adhesion and aggregation to form hemostasis plaque. Activation of prothrombin to the serine protease thrombin leads to converting fibrinogen into fibrin. Fibrin is then cross-linked by factor XIII to form a blood clot. Fibrin and fibronectin cross-link together and form a network that traps proteins and platelets, prevents further blood loss, facilitates cell migration, and provides a matrix scaffold for collagen deposition.

Platelets also release large amount of growth factors, cytokines, and proinflammatory factors such as serotonin, bradykinin, prostaglandins, prostacyclins, thromboxanes, and histamines. Thromboxanes and prostaglandins promote vasoconstriction to minimize blood loss, followed by vasodilation.

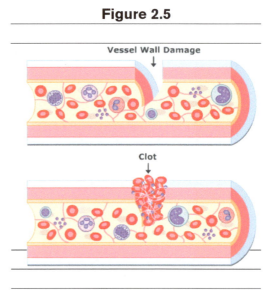

Figure 2.5

Schematic illustration of hemostasis

INFLAMMATORY RESPONSE

Cytokines present in the blood clot attract inflammatory cells, including polymorphonuclear leukocytes (PMNs) and macrophages, into the wound. PMNs are involved in phagocytosis and the clearance of debris, damaged cells, and bacteria. They also release large amount of inflammatory cytokines and growth factors. About two days after injury, macrophages replace PMNs and become the predominant cell type in the wound and continue to secrete major growth factors such as transforming growth factor-$\beta 1$ (TGF-$\beta 1$) and platelet drive growth factor (PDGF). In addition to phagocytosis and immune response, macrophages have been proposed to influence reepithelialization, granulation tissue formation, matrix deposition, and angiogenesis.

During the inflammatory phase, fibroblasts and endothelial cells release antibacterial superoxide in order to protect the wound from infection. In addition, superoxidase induces cell signaling for further stimulation of growth factor release. Taken together, the inflammatory response during wound healing provides pivotal conditions for resistance to wound infections and a bridge between the earlier phases of wound healing and the later stages when wound is repaired and stabilized.

Figure 2.6: Inflammation phase

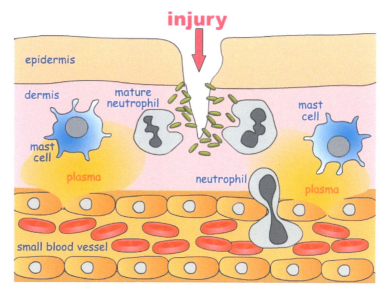

Schematic illustration of inflammatory response in dermal wound healing showing key inflammatory cells: mast cells and neutrophils

Courtesy of Birmingham City University—Faculty of Health Physiology

Figure 2.7: Wound healing phases and events

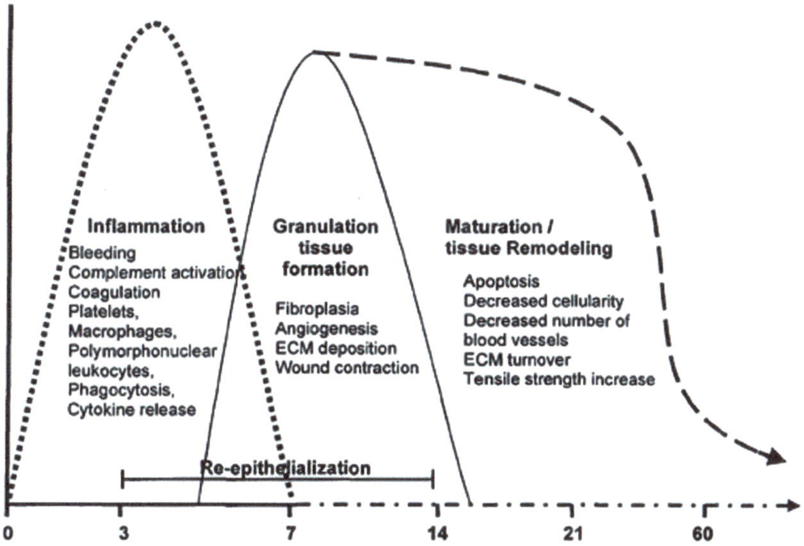

Healing is the interaction of a complex cascade of cellular events that generate the resurfacing, reconstitution, and restoration of the tensile strength of injured skin. Healing is a systematic process, traditionally explained in terms of three classic phases: inflammation, granulation tissue formation or proliferation, and maturation/tissue remodeling.

Days

REEPITHILIALIZATION

Immediately after injury, cytokines released from platelets activate keratinocytes. Migration of keratinocytes and hence reepithelialization starts as early as two hours after wounding. Growth factors such as keratinocyte growth factor (KGF) and epidermal growth factor (EGF) induce proliferation and migration of keratinocytes. The main sources of migrating keratinocytes during the reepithelialization process are basal keratinocytes from the wound edges, dermal appendages such as hair follicles, sweat glands and sebacious glands, and bone marrow−derived keratinocyte stem cells. Keratinocytes secrete proteases and plasminogen activators that activate plasmin, which dissolves the clot, the debris, and parts of the ECM and promotes cell migration.

The migration of keratinocytes over the wound site is also enhanced by lack of contact inhibition and nitric oxide released from PMNs, keratinocytes, and fibroblasts. Epithelial cells continue migrating across the wound bed until cells from different sides meet in the middle, at which point contact between keratinocytes inhibits further migration. Subsequently, new layers of keratinocytes differentiate and give rise to a stratified epidermis. Additionally, wound contraction by myofibroblasts present in the granulation tissue accelerates wound closure by bringing wound edges closer together. Fast keratinocyte migration and reepithelialization often leads to better wound healing outcomes and decreased scar formation. In contrast, exposure to air and/or lack of moisture retards the healing process. Keratinocytes are also involved in angiogenesis, matrix production, chemoattraction, and mitogenic activity by releasing vascular endothelial growth factor (VEGF), PDGF, and transforming growth factor-α (TGF-α).

GRANULATION TISSUE

The granulation tissue formation phase is characterized by fibroplasia in which the number of fibroblasts is increased in the wound. Soon after injury, local resident fibroblasts migrate into the wound site, undergo proliferation, and constitute the granulation tissue. The number of fibroblasts that are involved in phagocytosis and the deposition of new ECM in the wounded area peaks at one to two weeks postwounding, making them the dominant cell type in the granulation tissue. Depending on their origin, fibroblasts in the wound granulation tissue show phenotypically and functionally distinct characteristics that determine how they respond to wound-healing stimulation. Cells involved in the granulation tissue formation and wound healing are originated from different sources. For example, stem cells derived from muscle and adipose tissue, mesenchymal stem cell−like cells from surrounding healthy unwounded tissue, perivascular cells, and cells from the dermal sheath of the hair follicles have been suggested to contribute to granulation tissue formation.

Circulating blood-borne cells, such as fibrocytes that can differentiate into myofibroblasts, also populates granulation tissue. Fibrocytes also secrete angiogenic factors that induce neovascularization during wound healing. Pericytes and bone marrow−derived endothelial progenitor cells that enter to the blood circulation in response to cytokine released from the injury also integrate into the granulation tissue at the sites of new blood vessel growth. In addition, newly discovered, relatively poorly characterized blood-derived Dot cells that are believed to promote scarless dermal wound healing also migrate to wound, differentiate, and reside in the granulation tissue.

Similarities in the structure and cell populations of both skin and oral mucosa suggest that in both tissues progenitor cells involved in wound healing may be recruited from similar origins, with the exception that oral mucosa obviously lacks hair follicle–derived cells. Granulation tissue also contains increased number of inflammatory cells, such as macrophages and a provisional ECM that is mainly composed of fibronectin, type III collagen, glycosaminoglycans, proteoglycans, and hyaluronans.

The provisional matrix provides a hydrated matrix that facilitates the migration of cells to the granulation tissue. In addition, a low-oxygen environment stimulates neovascularization by inducing macrophages and platelets to secrete angiogenic factors such as fibronectin and increase growth factors that attract endothelial cells to the granulation tissue. Endothelial cells themselves secrete collagenases and plasminogen activators to degrade the clot ECM to facilitate their motility. Formation of new blood vessels continues increasingly in granulation tissue until after three to four weeks, when their number decreases through apoptosis.

Upon changes in ECM microenvironment caused by wounding, fibroblasts evolve into the protomyofibroblasts that will subsequently differentiate to myofibroblasts characterized by the expression of α-smooth muscle actin (α-SMA). Transition of fibroblasts to proto-myofibroblasts and to α-SMA-expressing myofibroblasts is thought to be regulated by extra domain A (EDA) fibronectin, growth factors such as TGF-β and PDGF, and by mechanical tension incurred from wounding and contraction. Myofibroblasts use α2β1 integrin to attach to collagen and pull collagen using actin-rich cytoskeleton that is linked to the cytoplasmic tail of α2β1 integrin. Therefore, in addition to the synthesis of ECM components, particularly type I collagen, myofibroblasts regulate wound contraction and ECM reorganization. Around after two weeks, soon after the formation of new epithelium over the granulation tissue, the number of myofibroblasts starts to decrease through apoptosis.

SKIN-TISSUE REMODELING

During wound healing, ECM components undergo substantial changes that include transition from clot of fibrin and fibronectin to a mixture of hyaluronate, proteoglycans, and collagen. Initially, collagen is deposited as a thin and randomly organized network that gradually is increased in thickness, rearranged, cross-linked, and aligned. This leads to the replacement of the provisional matrix with collagen-fiber bundles that more closely resemble normal unwounded tissue. During wound maturation and the tissue-remodeling phase, type III collagen, which is abundant during granulation tissue formation, is gradually degraded and type I collagen becomes dominant.

During several weeks to few months, as the remodeling phase progresses, the tensile strength of the wound increases with the strength reaching about 80% that of normal tissue. Depending on the size and location of the wound, the maturation phase can last from months to years after the injury. However, balance in the synthesis and degradation of collagen appears to be critical for a normal connective-tissue remodeling and ECM reorganization. For example, in gingiva the degradation and remodeling of collagen-rich ECM are essential in maintaining normal oral-mucosal connective tissue.

In vitro studies suggest that the uptake and lysosomal degradation of collagen by fibroblasts comprises a major pathway in the turnover of collagen and connective tissue remodeling. The uptake of collagen by fibroblasts involves the binding of collagen fibrils to the specific cell surface receptors. For example, phagocytosis of collagen by fibroblasts is mediated mostly by α2β1 integrin. In addition, urokinase-type plasminogen activator receptor associated protein (uPARAP)/Endo180, an endocytic receptor expressed on the cell surface, also binds to and mediates the endocytosis of collagen for lysosomal degradation, but its expression during wound healing is not known.

Matrix metalloproteinases (MMPs) released by fibroblasts cleave most of the ECM molecules and are also involved in the breakdown and remodeling during wound healing. Collagenases such as MMP1, MMP2, MMP8, MMP9, MMP13, and MMP14 that degrade connective-tissue collagen; gelatinases such as MMP2 and MMP9 that degrade basement membrane collagens; and stromelysins such as MMP3, MMP10, and MMP11 that degrade ECM proteoglycans, laminin, fibronectin, and gelatin play an important role in ECM turnover and remodeling during wound healing. Thus, abnormalities in MMP activity and/or the endocytosis or phagocytosis of ECM components may be associated with accumulation of excess collagen and scar formation.

Figure 2.8. Proliferative phases of wound healing

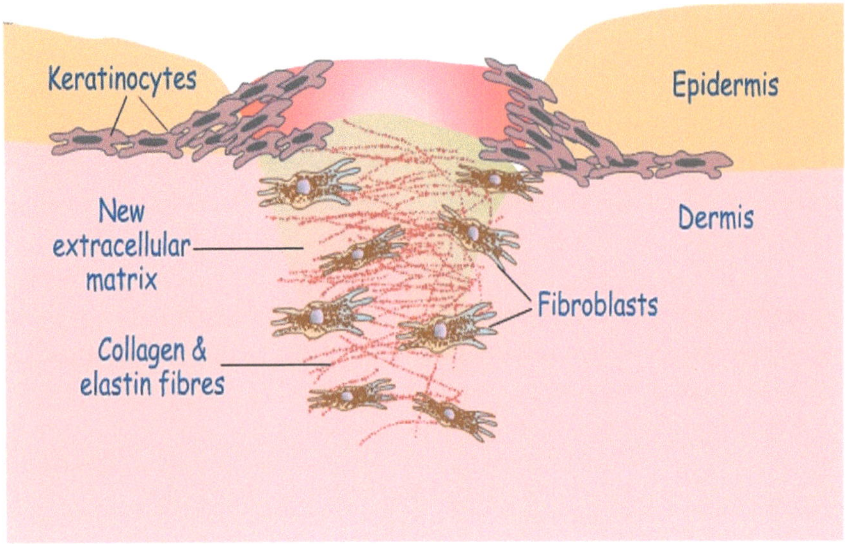

Schematic illustration of the proliferative phase of wound healing showing fibroblasts producing extracellular matrix and reepithelialization by keratinocytes

Courtesy of Birmingham City University—Faculty of Health Physiology

HAIR-GROWTH CYCLE

The three stages of the hair-growth cycles consist of a long growing phase or anagen, a brief transitional phase or catagen, and a short resting phase or telogen. The new cycle begins at the end of the resting phase when the hair falls out and a new hair starts growing in the follicle. Eyebrows and eyelashes have a growing phase of one to six months. Scalp hairs have a growing phase of two to six years. Under normal condition, it is estimated that about a hundred scalp hairs reach the end of the resting phase each day and fall out.

1. Anagen (growing) stage.

This is the name for the growing period of a hair follicle. The anagen stage for the hair follicles in the scalp typically lasts about three to five years.

2. Catagen (intermediate) stage.

At the end of the growth period, hair follicles prepare themselves for the resting phase. This transition period of a hair follicle from growth to rest is called the catagen stage. This stage of the hair growth cycle usually lasts about one to two weeks. During the catagen phase the deeper portions of the hair follicles start to collapse.

3. Telogen (resting or shedding) stage.

This is the resting period of a hair follicle. It is usually three to four months in length, and at the end of this period, older hairs that have finished their life will fall out and newer hairs will begin to grow. The growing (anagen) phase constitutes about 90% (a thousand days or more) of the growth cycle of a hair follicle, while the intermediate (catagen phase; ten days) and shedding (telogen phase; a hundred days) phases constitute only 10% of it. That is, at any given time, about 10% of hair follicles are in the intermediate and shedding phases; thus, not growing. These hair follicles, however, are randomly distributed over the scalp, so that no bald spots are seen.

Figure 2.9

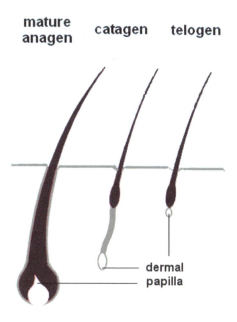

Schematic illustration of the hair growth cycle

HAIR DISORDERS

Hair disorders include hair loss (alopecia), excessive hairiness (hirsutism), ingrown beard hairs (pseudofolliculitis barbae), and hair-shaft disorders that are due to overprocessed hair coloring, permanent waves, excessive heating, or certain diseases. Most hair disorders are benign and not serious, but they are often undesirable due to, foremost, cosmetic concerns that necessitate their treatment.

HAIR LOSS (ALOPECIA)

Alopecia is a disorder in which the hair falls out from skin areas where it is usually present, such as the scalp and body. This loss interferes with the many useful biologic functions of the hair, including sun protection (mainly to the scalp) and the spreading of sweat gland products. Hair loss has psychological impact in the individual. Patients with hair loss can suffer tremendously from social withdrawal. Nonscarring alopecia may involve hair loss all over or in circular areas, a receding hairline, broken hairs, a smooth scalp, inflammation, and possibly loss of lashes, eyebrows, or pubic hair.

Nonscarring alopecia may be caused by skin disorders or certain diseases, certain drugs, autoimmune disease, iron deficiency, severe stress, scalp radiation, pregnancy, or pulling at your own hair. Scarring alopecia is limited to particular areas. Symptoms are inflammation at the edge of and follicle loss toward the center of lesions, violet-colored skin abnormalities, and scaling. Skin disorders, diseases, or bacterial infections can cause scarring alopecia.

EXCESSIVE HAIRINESS (HIRSUTISM)

Hirsutism is male-pattern hair growth in women, which is usually accompanied by irregular menstruation, lack of ovulation, acne, deepening of voice, balding, and genital abnormalities. Symptoms of hair-shaft disorders are split ends and hair that is dry, brittle, and coarse, as well as skin and other abnormalities. Excess of androgen, a steroid hormone that stimulates the development of male sex organs and secondary sexual characteristics, is considered as a main etiology of hirsutism. This overproduction of androgen could result from certain drugs or conditions.

MELANOCYTES AND SKIN COLOR

The epidermis also contains melanocytes, which are cells that produce a skin pigment called melanin. Melanin is a substance that gives the skin and hair its natural color. In humans, those with darker skin have higher amounts of melanin. Melanin absorbs the sun's radiation energy and protects the skin from the detrimental effects of ultraviolet rays.

Melanin is stored in cell organelles called melanosomes. In hot areas with higher exposure to solar radiation, the ratio of melanocytes to keratinocytes is about 1:4. In contrast, in colder areas with less daily sunlight, the ratio may be as low as 1:30. Main factors that contribute to the stimulation of melanin production may be sun exposure, melanocyte-stimulating hormones (MSH), adrenocorticotropic hormones (ACTH), estrogens, and progesterones. As people age, the number of melanocytes populating the skin is substantially declined.

Figure 2.10

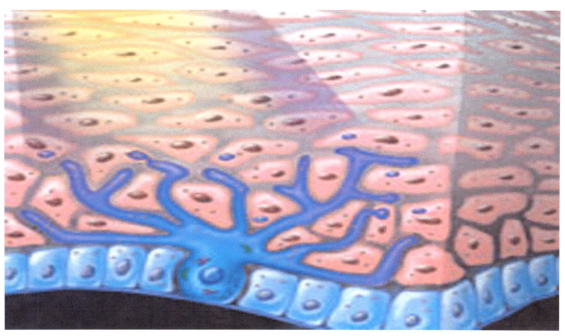

illustration by Matt Hazzard

Melanocytes (dark blue cells) distribute pigment, also known as melanin. Keratinocytes (light blue cells) make up 90% of skin cells, and as the keratinocytes are pushed up to the surface by new cells beneath them, the melanin gets more and more concentrated. Skin is rich in one type of melanin, called eumelanin, that absorbs the UV light before it can get down to the danger zone—where the melanocytes live. Skin cancer happens when UV light mutates cells in the danger zone.

NAILS

The nail consists of dead cells pushed outward by dividing cells in the root, a fold of epidermis at the base of the nail. Fingernails and toenails are made of a hard protein called keratin. Along with hair, they are an appendage of the skin. The nail consists of the nail plate, the matrix, the nail bed, and the surrounding grooves. If the root is destroyed, the nail ceases to grow. One cycle of growth from root to tip is achieved in about four months. The small-celled and relatively bloodless tissue near the base of the nail forms a white, crescent-shaped spot called the lunula or moon.

No pigment occurs in nail cells, but since they are translucent, their appearance is pink because of blood vessels beneath. Nail disorders can result from infections, injuries, internal diseases such as certain lung diseases (which can cause yellow-nail syndrome), and structural complications such as an ingrown toenail. With aging, nails become dry, brittle, and flat or concave instead of convex. They may develop ridges along their length. Nail color may change to yellow or gray. Brittle nails may split.

Toenails require special attention in older people and in people with diabetes or peripheral vascular disease. Infections may involve the nail itself, the bed under the nail, or the skin around the nail. Most nail infections are fungal, but bacterial and viral infections can also occur. Bacterial infections such as onychomycosis and paronychia may occur in the cuticle or nail folds.

Figure 2.11: Basic nail anatomy

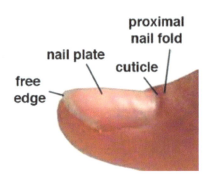

chapter 3

Nutrition and Skin Rejuvenation

THE ROLE OF NUTRITION

BEST DIET FOR THE SKIN

MAGIC OF A BALANCED DIET

FLUIDS, FRUITS, AND VEGETABLES

HIGH-PROTEIN DIET AND HEALTHY SKIN

VITAMIN MINERALS AND SKIN REJUVENATION

VITAMIN A

VITAMIN C

VITAMIN B COMPLEX

VITAMIN D

VITAMIN E

SUDDEN WEIGHT LOSS AND SKIN SAGGING

BAD DIET AND SKIN WRINKLING

CHAPTER 3

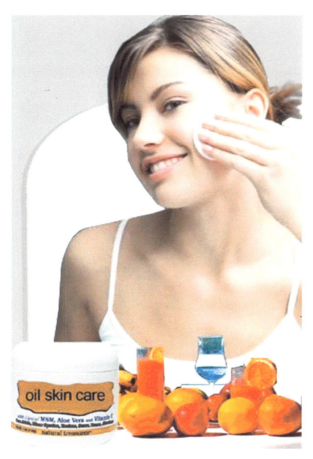

Nutrition and Skin Rejuvenation

THE ROLE OF NUTRITION

Some people consider nutrition to be far less effective for skin health and rejuvenation than undergoing cosmetic plastic surgery. On the other hand, others believe that nutrition makes a significant difference. Eating healthy and proper foods can effectively contribute to the skin freshness and rejuvenation. Food supplement and vitamin companies advertise selling skin pills that they claim rejuvenate the skin in a short period of time. The question whether or not eating habit has a scientifically proven role in making a difference in skin rejuvenation warrants considerable research. The fact is, shifting to new nutrition habits and particular diets are less likely to diminish all wrinkles or totally slow down the skin aging. However, several pieces of evidence indicate that nutrition and proper diet cannot be without any effect on the skin. Health food and vegetables affect every organ in the body, and skin is no exception. Therefore, while a skin cream may provide a number of important ingredients with scientifically proven effects, it would not be sufficient to guarantee proper skin nutrition.

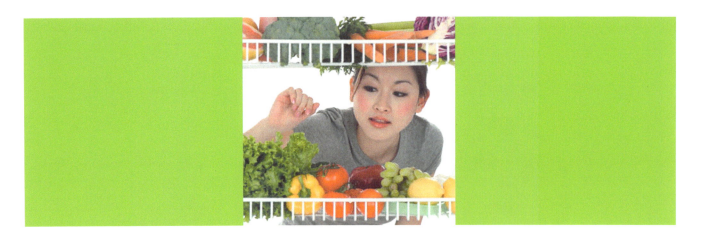

Cells in the human body require multiple nutrients and metabolites such as vitamins, minerals, and essential amino acids that can be obtained only from healthy foods and fresh vegetables. When the nutrients are ingested and absorbed into the bloodstream, it is ensured that they will be delivered to the skin cells. Provided healthy and proper nourishment, the human body can produce many essential molecules for different organs, including skin. Therefore, the consensus is that no skin cream or lotion can replace a good diet. The effectiveness of the ingredients in a skin cream or lotion depends on the skin's condition, the concentration of the ingredients, the manufacturing technology, and a good nutrition. Applying a lotion with nutrients to the surface of skin does not guarantee that those nutrients essentially infiltrate into skin cells. This means that a combination of factors such as applying topical skin creams, skin hygiene, and a good diet that provides vitamins and other necessary nutrients for the skin can achieve satisfactory results in a skin-rejuvenation program.

BEST DIET FOR THE SKIN

It is generally accepted that the diet optimal for overall health can be most favorable for skin health too, but one needs to set a balanced diet carefully in order to reach optimal conditions for the skin. Generally, a balanced diet refers to an eating paradigm that possesses all necessary nutrients within a best possible range. This range is carefully planned in such a way to prevent vitamin and/or mineral deficiencies and/or protein malnutrition. However, in order to achieve the maximum antiaging effects, one may have to eat some nutrients in greater amounts than those found in a basic balanced diet. The simplest to remain on a balanced diet is to have a daily adequate quantity of fruits and vegetables while staying within energy needs.

MAGIC OF A BALANCED DIET

To make sure that all necessary nutrients are given to the body in sufficient quantities, a wide variety of fruits and vegetables on a daily basis must be ingested. A balanced diet contains all five vegetable subgroups, including dark-green vegetables, orange vegetables, legumes, starchy vegetables, and other miscellaneous vegetables for several times a week. Having three cups per day of low-fat milk or equivalent milk products is a must in a balanced diet program. In addition, at least three-ounce equivalents of whole grain products per day, with the rest of the recommended grains coming from enriched or whole-grain products, should be in the daily uptake.

Figure 3.1

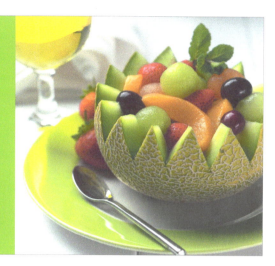

Dietary experts recommend that every person should eat at least five servings of fresh fruits and vegetables every day. Increasing daily consumption of fruits and vegetables is one of the easiest changes that can be made to increase the level of overall health, including skin freshness.

FLUIDS, FRUITS, AND VEGETABLES

Drinking ample amounts of fluids during the day to some extent makes the skin less prone to developing of wrinkles. Drinking pure water and fresh and natural fruit juice ensures proper hydration of the body and reduces skin dehydration. Drinking six to eight glasses of water a day is usually recommend. Having coffee and sodas that contain caffeine, a diuretic ingredient, makes people urinate more often and lose more water. Drinking too much fluid before going to bed may cause morning puffiness and notably stretch the skin. Consumption of fresh fruits and vegetables in abundant quantities is desirable for the skin health.

In particular, fruits and vegetables not only provide a lot of fluid needed for the body, but they are also critical for preventing early skin aging because they contain a wide variety of antioxidants. These antioxidants save skin cells from the harmful effect of free radicals, which are out of control due to exposure to environmental factors of the skin. In order to make sure fruits and vegetables have all their antioxidants intact, they must be fresh and uncooked. Since heat inactivates most antioxidants, if cooked vegetables are desired, they must be only minimally cooked. Cooking with high temperature causes an exponential boost in the rate of chemical reactions, leading to increased degradation and oxidation of nutrients.

The content of free radicals increases dramatically as well when food is cooked with extreme heat. As a result, less essential nutrients and more aging-promoting free radicals are consumed. Taken together, reducing cooking time and avoiding deep-frying, grilling, and cooking with small amounts of oil or fat can make a difference in your skin health and overall wellness.

HIGH-PROTEIN DIET AND HEALTHY SKIN

Besides water, protein is the most abundant component in human body. Approximately 10% of the total protein occurs in the skin. Lack of protein and a fat-free diet may negatively impact the health of the skin. Protein is the basic building block of blood, bone, muscles, cartilage, skin, hair, and fingernails. It is an important component of enzymes necessary for biochemical reactions and hormones and plays a pivotal role in the red blood cells in the form of hemoglobin to transfer oxygen. Therefore, a good dietcan directly influence blood-cell function and, in general, overall health and can provide essential elements to keep the skin healthy and fresh. Proteins are made from the combination of more than twenty amino acids, nine of which are not produced by the body and must be obtained through the diet. An average adult male and female must have at least 57 g and 48 g, respectively, of protein in their daily diet.

Foods that are high in protein include beef, chicken, fish, turkey, lamb, milk, white cheese, yogurt, cottage cheese, cream cheese, eggs, peanut butter (with bread or crackers), dried beans, and peas (with bread, cornbread, rice).

Figure 3.2

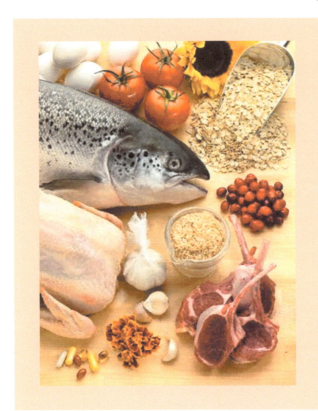

Protein is required by the body for the growth, maintenance, and repair of all cells. High-protein foods help you feel physically and emotionally fit, lose weight, and keep the body (including skin) healthy.

VITAMINS, MINERALS, AND SKIN REJUVENATION

Vitamins and minerals are essential for the proper function of the skin. Insufficiencies of some minerals and vitamins are specifically unfavorable to the skin and may accelerate its aging or lead to other dermal diseases. To increase the efficiency of any skin-rejuvenation diet, having adequate but optimal quantities of vitamins and minerals is crucial. This means not only having excessive vitamin and mineral supplement doses do not provide extra benefits but also, as the matter of fact, might be toxic to the cells. For vitamins, one should not exceed safety limits and must follow a recommended daily allowance in order to acquire the maximum benefits. In this section, vitamins and minerals that are particularly important for skin health and rejuvenation are discussed.

VITAMIN A

Vitamin A, also called retinol, helps eyes adjust to light changes. It also maintains the moisture of the eyes, skin, and mucosal membranes. Vitamin A is critical for the normal life cycle of skin cells. It is suggested that a lack of vitamin A may lead to skin dryness and fragility and the development of wrinkles. It is now conceivable that in people with vitamin A deficiency, any skin-treatment program may be not fully effective. The daily recommended dosage of vitamin A for women is 800 mcg and for men 1000 mcg. Important sources of vitamin A in foods include beef liver, egg yolk, cheddar cheese, and milk. Carrots or broccoli supply carotenoids that can be converted into vitamin A in the body. Excessive vitamin A ingestion may produce severe toxicity.

VITAMIN C

Vitamin C, also known as ascorbic acid, is necessary for wound healing. It prevents cell damage, promotes healthy gingiva and teeth, and strengthens the immune system. Vitamin C is a required element for the synthesis of collagen, a key structural protein in the skin. Deficiency of vitamin C reduces skin flexibility and its capacity to heal. Vitamin C is abundant in fresh fruits and vegetables, particularly in citrus products, tomatoes, berries, potatoes, green and red peppers, broccoli, and spinach.

Figure 3.3

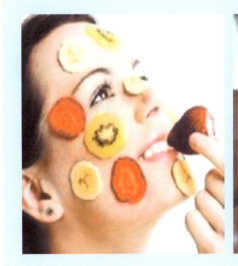
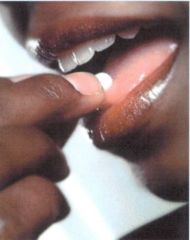

To date, a number of studies show that certain vitamins and minerals, when taken internally, can positively influence skin appearance, beauty, and overall health.

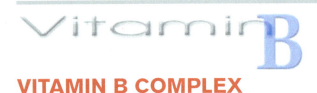

VITAMIN B COMPLEX

The family of B-complex vitamins includes vitamins B1 (thiamine), B2 (riboflavin), B3 (niacin), B5 (pantothenate), B6 (pyridoxine), B12 (cyancobalamin), and folate. B1 vitamin is necessary for adrenal gland function, proper immune performance, and the synthesis of neurotransmitters. It also plays a role in the metabolism of food and alcohol.

B2 is required for energy production and oxygen utilization. The symptoms of low B2 include fatigue, blindness, and anemia. Crusting around the mouth can also be seen in B2 deficiency. Lack of vitamins B1 and B2 may lead to the development of special forms of dermatitis. Mild deficiencies may not be noticed but may still lead to some extent of skin damage. People who consume a diet based mainly on processed grains are particularly prone to developing B1 and B2 insufficiency.

B3 is necessary for the body's production of energy. It is also recommended for people who suffer high cholesterol, schizophrenia, neurological disease, and Raynaud's syndrome. B5 is sometimes referred to as the "antistress" vitamin. It is also necessary for the proper function of our immune system and adrenal stress hormone production.

B6 and folic acid together regulate homocysteine levels. Homocysteine is a derivative of protein breakdown that damages arteries and contribute to cholesterol deposits. Folic acid deficiencies have been linked to birth defects. Women on birth control pills, pregnant women, patients with heart disease, and people taking antibiotics must take between 400–800 mcg of folic acid per day.

B12 is essential for a variety of synthetic processes in the cells, including normal gene function, energy production, the formation of blood cells, and proper immunity. The deficiency of B12 vitamin is particularly harmful to neurons and rapidly dividing cells, including skin cells. Mild B12 deficiency is often undiagnosed and shows no obvious symptoms. However, it has been reported that depression may occur in B12 deficiency. B12 vitamin is found in meat, poultry, fish, eggs, and dairy products. Absorption of vitamin B12 requires a protein produced by the stomach called intrinsic factor. Lack of intrinsic factor due to the atrophy of stomach glands and certain autoimmune diseases may lead to reduced absorption of B12. For people whose B12 deficiency is due to poor absorption, the vitamin must to be taken by nasal spray or via injection.

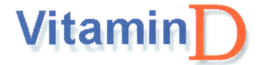

Vitamin D is a fat-soluble vitamin. It is a powerful antioxidant and anticarcinogen. There are numerous benefits of vitamin D for the skin and overall health. Vitamin D is essential for the formation of healthy and strong teeth, bones, and nails. It also helps for the proper absorption of calcium by the body and the regulation of calcium and phosphorus levels in the blood. In addition, vitamin D improves the absorption of vitamin A and C. Calciferol is the main proform of the vitamin D. It is converted into an active form in the liver and kidneys once produced or ingested. Vitamin D can ameliorate skin cancer, heart disease, diabetes, and other health and skin problems. The main source of vitamin D is simply exposure to sunlight. Ultraviolet light from sun's radiation acts on skin, providing no sunscreen is used, and allows it to synthesize vitamin D. However, prolonged sun exposure may lead to skin cancer and premature skin aging.

Figure 3.4

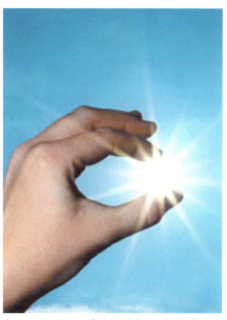

The main source of vitamin D is exposure of the skin to sunlight radiation, providing no sunscreen is used. Prolonged sun exposure may lead to skin cancer and premature skin aging.

Five to ten minutes of daily summer sun exposure on face, hands, arms, and back will provide enough ultraviolet light exposure to produce the required amount of vitamin D for the body. Dark-skinned individuals need longer periods of sun exposure. In the areas with less sun radiation, careful attention must be paid into the diet in order to achieve the adequate levels of vitamin D required for the body.

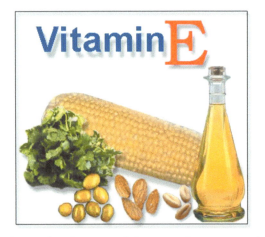

Vitamin E is a principal fat-soluble antioxidant vitamin in the body. It protects cellular membranes and lipoproteins. Both oral consumption and topical administration of vitamin E are substantially effective on the maintenance of the unsaturated fatty acids in the skin-cell membranes. Topical skin products that contain vitamin E have become an essential part of healthy skin care. Free radicals are believed to promote skin aging, and skin care products that contain antioxidants can effectively influence skin health and rejuvenation. Because of its antioxidant property, vitamin E is crucial in protecting skin cells from ultraviolet light, pollution, drugs, and other elements that produce cell-damaging free radicals. To obtain maximum benefit when applying products containing vitamin E, it is recommended to use cream or lotions that contain the vitamin in its natural alcohol form (alpha-tocopherol). The acetate form (alpha-tocopherol acetate) of vitamin E is a less effective antioxidant.

The benefits of vitamin E for healthy skin care also include its ability to regulate vitamin A in the body, which itself is important for healthy skin. Both orally taken vitamin E and supplemented in lotions, creams, or other skin care products may be synergistic in implementing the antiaging effect on skin. Vitamin E lotions can prevent sunburns by protecting the epidermis layer of the skin from the destructive effects of ultraviolet light; therefore, vitamin E added to sunscreens may increase their efficacy.

Sunblocks enriched with vitamin E must be administered several minutes before exposure to the sun radiation in order to allow for proper penetration of the vitamin into the epidermis layer. Topical administration of vitamin E also recommended for the treatment of psoriasis. Intake of vitamin E by mouth is prescribed for the treatment of erythema, an inflammation of skin that manifests reddish, painful, and sensitive skin bumps. Other benefits of vitamin E for skin care include reduction of stretch marks and age spots, enhancement of the skin's barrier function, maintenance of the skin's oil balance, and prevention of water loss from skin.

SUDDEN WEIGHT LOSS AND SKIN SAGGING

One of the most undesirable conditions that increase the development of wrinkles is the frequent gaining and losing of weight. Gaining weight and accumulation of excess fat make the skin stretch in order to accommodate the space needed for the new fat deposits. Upon sudden weight reduction or loss of the very same body fat, skin crumples up and becomes droopy. This condition is known as sagginess of the skin. The extent of skin sagging depends on the extent of the weight loss, age, gender, and heredity. Sequential gaining and losing of weight may have damaging effects not only on the skin but also on the overall health. In addition, upon aging over time, the skin's supporting structure tends to break down leading to loss of skin youthful appearance. Combination of this with genetic factors, hormonal changes, and sun damage may promote the skin to sag and hang.

Figure 3.5

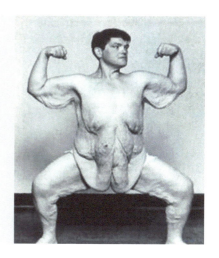

Skin sagging due to sudden weight loss

Sagging and loose skin is usually a sign of aging. However, many people can face this problem even at a young age due to sudden weight loss.

The best way to prevent skin sagging is to implement proper skin care strategies and a balanced diet. Fruits and vegetables and foods rich in omega-3 fatty acids, like fish oil or cod oil in the diet, can help to prevent skin from sagging. It is suggested that drinking plenty of water and regular exercising can also help maintain skin elasticity and retard the manifestation of wrinkles and fine lines. Massaging the skin with natural oils such as vitamin E, coconut, and almond oil contributes to the moisturizing of the skin and increases its elasticity to prevent sagging. Excessive exposure to sunlight can cause skin sagging and wrinkles. Protection form UV light by using sunscreens or sunblocks may substantially reduce the skin aging.

BAD DIET AND SKIN WRINKLING

Several reports have suggested that increased ingestion of olive oil, olives, fish, reduced-fat milk, milk products, eggs, nuts, legumes, vegetables, whole-grain cereals, fruit, fruit products, tea, and water may reduce skin wrinkling. However, even though not scientifically proven, skin aging and wrinkling in the elderly has been linked to higher than normal intakes of saturated fat, red meat, high-in-fat dairy products, soft drinks, cakes, pastries, desserts, potatoes, butter, and margarine. This dietary information should not be taken as an established fact for avoiding certain types of food. Several other variables should be taken into the consideration before starting a diet program to battle skin aging.

Figure 3.6. Signs of bad diets

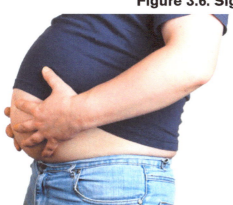

Signs of bad diet include low energy/fatigue, feeling down/depressed, premenstrual syndrome, constant hunger, bingeing and craving, irritability, anxiety, mental fogginess.

chapter 4

Most Common Skin Problems

RATIONALE

DRY AND ROUGH SKIN

TREATMENT OF DRY SKIN

OIL-PRONE SKIN

TREATMENT OF OIL-PRONE SKIN

DIET FOR OIL-PRONE SKIN

SWEATING DISORDERS

CAUSE OF SWEAT ODOR

DIMINISHED SWEATING

HYPERHIDROSIS (EXCESSIVE SWEATING)

TREATMENT OF HYPERHIDROSIS

MILIARIA (PRICKY HEAT)

SUN-DAMAGED SKIN

PROTECTION FROM UV RAYS

DARK UNDEREYE CIRCLES

AGING, SAGGING SKIN

ETIOLOGY OF SAGGING SKIN

NATURAL SKIN AGING

BIOLOGY OF SKIN AGING

SMOKING AND SKIN AGING

LACK OF EXERCISE AND SKIN AGING

REACTIVE OXYGEN SPECIES (ROS) AND SKIN AGING

EXTREME HOT OR COLD WEATHER

STRESS AND ALCOHOL CONSUMPTION

STRETCH MARKS

TREATMENT OF STRETCH MARKS

SCAR FORMATION

CELLULITES

TREATMENT OF CELLULITES

PIGMENTATION DISORDERS (VITILIGO)

HYPERPIGMENTATION

MELASMA AND CHOLASMA

TREATMENT OF MELASMA

MOLES

ROSACEA

ROSACEA SUBTYPES

ACNE VULGARIS

CAUSES OF ACNE

TYPES AND STAGES OF ACNE

TREATMENT OF ACNE

ACNE MEDICATION

TECHNIQUES FOR ACNE CONTROL

DIET AND ACNE PROGRESSION

AGGRAVATION OF ACNE

ACNE SCARS

TREATMENT FOR ACNE SCARS

SPIDER VEINS

SCLEROTHERAPY

LASER TREATMENT FOR SPIDER VEINS

ALOPECIA (HAIR LOSS)

HIRSUTISM (EXCESSIVE FEMALE HAIR GROWTH)

TREATMENT OF HIRSUTISM

PSEUDOFOLLICULITIS BARBAE (INGROWN BEARD HAIRS)

ADVANCED SKIN CARE STRATEGIES

CHAPTER 4

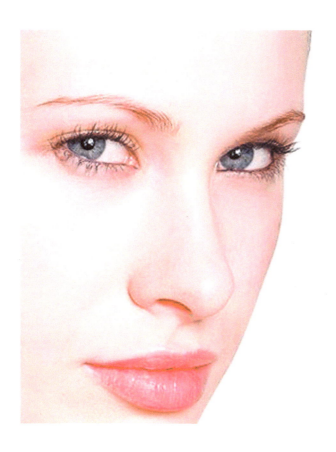

Most Common Skin Problems

RATIONALE

A precise understanding of the multiple factors governing skin behavior and the technical means of identifying them is necessary to establish a scientific skin care approach. In order to achieve this goal a medical aesthetician must be aware of skin types and treatment protocols. In this chapter, the most common skin problems that affect the skin and likely result is health, social, and behavioral concerns are discussed.

DRY AND ROUGH SKIN

Figure 4.1. Dry skin

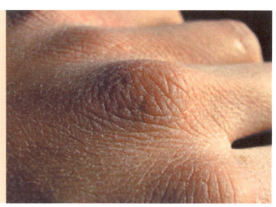

Dry skin is most common in lower legs, arms, flanks (sides of the abdomen), and thighs. The symptoms most often associated with dry skin include scaling, itching, and cracks in the skin.

In contrast to oil-prone skin, dry skin becomes dehydrated and rough since the oil glands are hypoactive and do not supply enough lubrication to the skin. Dry skin has a low level of sebum and can be prone to sensitivity. The skin may have a desiccated appearance caused by lack of moisture. It usually feels tight and uncomfortable after washing unless some type of moisturizer or skin cream is applied. Dry skin in some individuals may appear tedious, especially on the cheeks and around the eyes.

Symptoms of extremely dry, dehydrated skin can be manifested as chapping and cracking of the skin. Dryness can be worsened by wind, high temperature, and prolonged exposure to air-conditioning. Dry skins tend to flake, chap, and feel tight. Usually skin becomes rough, scaly, and prone to fine wrinkles, age spots, and loss of elasticity. Causes of dry skin vary, but most common causes include heredity, poor diet (especially deficiencies of vitamin A and the B vitamins), environmental factors (such as exposure to sun, wind, cold), underactive thyroid, and diabetes. In addition, chemicals, cosmetics, or excessive washing with harsh soaps can result in dry skin. Furthermore, conditions such as dermatitis, eczema, psoriasis or seborrhea, and certain drugs—including diuretics, antispasmodics, and antihistamines—can contribute to dry skin.

TREATMENT OF DRY SKIN

Due to deposits, cleansing dry skin using tap water can be too harsh. Hot water for washing the dry skin is also not recommended. Particularly for the face, using mineral water is a better choice. Washing dry skin with excess commercial soap and water removes the natural oils that protect the skin. Coming in contact with highly alkaline soaps and detergents like washing sodas and powders, which contain high alkaline and drying ingredients, can aggravate the dryness and must be avoided.

Dry skin needs ample of light but careful cleansing, regular stimulation with massage, and openhanded amounts of oil and moisturizing lotion. A moisturizer increases the water content of the outer layers of the skin and gives it a reduced dryness and softer appearance. Washcloth with a rough texture can irritate the skin. Applying a spray of mineral water on the face on a regular basis can reduce the irritation. People with dry skin must use nondetergent neutral-pH products to cleanse their skin. Applying baby oil gently after a bath or a shower can improve the skin condition.

OIL-PRONE SKIN

In individuals with oil-prone skin, excess oil is produced by skin hyperactive oil glands. Oily skin looks shiny, thick, and dull colored. In this type of skin, the oil-producing sebaceous glands are overactive and produce more oil than is needed. If not cleansing, excess secreted oil may give a saturated, greasy, and shiny appearance to the skin. Often, chronically oily skin has coarse pores and pimples and unpleasant blemishes. The pores are enlarged, and the skin has a coarse appearance. The goal is to control the release of oil, hydrate, minimize pores, and improve the blemishes. The most common causes of oily skin include heredity, imbalanced diet, changes in hormone levels, pregnancy, birth control pills, cosmetics, humidity, and hot weather. The only advantage of oily skin is that it ages at a slower rate than other skin types.

TREATMENT OF OIL-PRONE SKIN

Oily skin needs special cleansing with abundance of hot water and soap to prevent the pores from being clogged. However, people with oily skin should avoid heavy cleansing creams, cleansers that strip the skin excessively off, and strong soaps that may cause flakiness. Excessive or harsh cleansing can cause a reaction known as reactive seborrhea, in which the oil glands are restimulated to compensate for the washed off natural oil.

Thus, more oil is produced and released on the skin surface. Cleansers or lotions that contain alcohol are not the best selections for oil-prone skins. Products that make the skin stretch tight and dehydrated should not be used. They cause the upper layers of the skin to shrink, leading to restriction of oil flow through the pores, blockages, and breakouts. Using a pure soap with no artificial additives and an antibacterial cleansing lotion or a medicated soap in combination with a water rich in minerals tremendously improve the condition of oily prone skin. Hot water dissolves skin oil better than lukewarm or cold water.

Rubbing soap into the skin can clog pores. In order to cleanse oily skin, oil-based products are recommended as they effectively dissolve sebum. While people with oil-prone skin must keep their skin very clean, washing the face should be limited to two or three times a day. Frequent washing may stimulate the skin to produce more oil. However, if the skin is extremely oily, three or four daily cleansings, but little or no moisturizing may be applied. After cleansing, using a natural oil-free moisturizer helps to keep the skin agile. When cleansing, it is a good practice to massage the face with fingertips by an upward and outward motion. If applying cosmetic and facial care products, those which are specifically designed for oily skin must be used. Before applying makeup, an antiseptic day cream with active ingredients such as benzyl peroxide, which reduces sebaceous secretions, is recommended.

DIET FOR OIL-PRONE SKIN

A diet rich in proteins but restricted in fat, sugar, fluids, and salt may be a diet of choice for people with oil-prone skin. Leafy green vegetables and fresh fruits are highly recommended. Consumption of pork, fried and seasoned foods, any oils that have been subjected to heat, and soft drinks or alcoholic beverages may aggravate oily skin. Surprisingly, even a slight deficiency in vitamin B2 can cause and/or intensify oily skin. Administration of necessary vitamins, iron, and similar substances can be considered as effective dietary strategies to ameliorate oily skin. Buckwheat, black beans, and whole rice are excellent sources of iron. Drinking plenty of soft water keeps the skin hydrated and contributes to detoxification that could be helpful in reducing skin oil.

Figure 4.2. Oil-prone skin

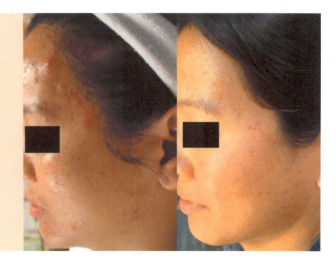

Oily skin is characterized by pros and cons. Oily skin provides natural protection from wrinkles and prevents it from drying out, but sometimes overproduction of oil can lead to clogged pores and ultimately acne.

SWEATING DISORDERS

Sweat is made by sweat glands and carried to the skin's surface by sweat ducts. Sweat consists primarily of water, sodium chloride, odurants 2- and 4-methylphenol, and a small amount of urea. Sweating is primarily a means of thermoregulation to keep the body cool. It is believed that sweating helps the body to remove toxins; however, this warrants further scientific research. Evaporation of sweat from the skin surface has a cooling effect, and hence, people sweat more when it is warm. Sweating also occurs under stress or exercise. Hypohidrosis, or diminished sweating, and hyperhidrosis, or excessive sweating, are two common sweating disorders that must be carefully monitored and treated in order to keep normal perspiration in a balanced state.

CAUSE OF SWEAT ODOR

Sweat glands are divided into two types: apocrine and eccrine. Apocrine glands can be found over the entire body and produce a salt-mitigated sweat in response to increased body temperature. The sweat is normally odorless unless normal flora bacteria that are present on the skin get the opportunity to decay the sweat within an hour. The apocrine glands' odor can also become offensive after consumption of spicy food, such as garlic and curry, alcohol, or certain medications. On the other hand, eccrine glands can be found most commonly in the underarms, breasts, and the area between thighs and abdomen. Eccrine glands produce a thick secretion that contains pheromones.

DIMINISHED SWEATING

Diminished sweating is usually limited to a specific area of the body. It can be caused by a skin injury, radiation, bacterial infection, inflammation, or by a connective tissue disease such as scleroderma and systemic lupus erythematosus. In addition, it has been suggested that in Sjögren's syndrome the sweat glands may be damaged and lead to diminished sweating. Sjögren's syndrome is an autoimmune disease characterized by dryness of the mouth and eyes. It is characterized by the abnormal production of antibodies that cause invasive inflammation in lachrymal and salivary glands that are responsible for producing tears and saliva, respectively.

Patients with this disease suffer from dry eyes, dry mouth, and probably dry, heated, blushed, and sensitive skin. Diminished sweating may also be due to drugs, especially those that have anticholinergic effects. Individuals with diminished sweating may be prone to severe heatstroke. Lack of sweating over a large portion of the body may cause overheat. The best and quickest treatment is exposure to cooling systems, such as air-conditioning and wearing wet garments.

HYPERHIDROSIS (EXCESSIVE SWEATING)

People with hyperhidrosis or excessive sweating may sweat constantly and abundantly. This condition may cause anxiety, leading to social withdrawal. Unfortunately, people suffering from excessive sweating tend to sweat even without conditions such as fever or exposure to very warm environments. Excessive sweating may occur on the entire surface of the skin; however, it can be more often seen in the palms of the hands, the soles of the feet, the armpits, or the genital area. Severe, chronic sweating can make the affected area red, inflamed, wrinkled, and cracked. The areas with excessive sweating are also prone to fungal and microbial infection due to prolonged wetness, heat, and lack of exposure to natural light. Bromhidrosis is a condition of abnormal or unpleasant body odor due to apocrine gland secretion and the breakdown of sweat components by bacteria and yeasts that are normally present on the skin.

Figure 4.3. Excessive sweating

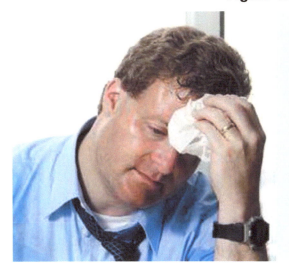

About 2% of the world's population endures excessive sweating. It can be the result of diseases (such as lung and spinal cord problems), improper glucose levels, tuberculosis, or hormonal changes. Physical activity, emotional and social factors, overworking of the nervous system, and dieting habits can also cause excessive sweating.

TREATMENT OF HYPERHIDROSIS

Excessive sweating can be controlled to some degree with commercial antiperspirants. However, stronger treatments are often needed, especially for the palms, soles, armpits, or genital area. Applying commercially available solutions that contain methenamine or aluminum chloride may be partially effective. For maximum effect, the sweaty area should be dried before applying the solution twice a day. Orally taken drugs such as phenoxybenzamine and propantheline are also prescribed for control of excessive sweating. Treatment with the injection of botulinum toxin (Botox) into the affected area is also very effective.

Botox temporally paralyzes the smooth muscles that are responsible for contracting the sweat glands and dramatically reduces their secretions. The effect of Botox remains for up to three to four months, when another injection of the drug is required to boost up its effect. If drugs are not effective to cure excessive sweating, the patient may choose to undergo an invasive surgical procedure that involves removing a part of skin from affected area containing nerves that control the sweat glands.

However, direct excision of the axillary skin or neurosurgical sympathectomy for hyperhidrosis of the affected skin creates unwanted and unattractive scarring, often with prolonged recovery and limitation of movement. Excessive sweating limited to the armpits is sometimes treated by liposuction to remove the sweat glands. Frequent cleansing with soap and water helps to remove the microbial agents that aggravate odor. Cleansing with an antiseptic soap containing clindamycin or erythromycin may be highly effective. Shaving the hair in the armpits may also help control the odor.

MILIARIA (PRICKLY HEAT)

Miliaria or prickly heat is an irritating skin rash caused by trapped sweat. Prickly heat occurs when the sweat gland ducts that carry the sweat to the surface of skin get congested or blocked. The trapped sweat causes inflammation along with irritation, itchiness, and very tiny swellings. However, prickly heat can also be manifested as large and blushed areas of skin. Prickly heat mostly occurs in geographic areas with warm and humid climates. Prickly heat onset is frequently seen on the skin where two parts of the body touch each other, such as under the breasts, on the inner thighs, and under the arms. Use of powders, antiperspirants, and keeping the skin cool and dry can minimize the chance of conditions that contribute to prickly heat manifestation. Corticosteroid creams or lotions may be helpful in alleviating the symptoms.

Figure 4.4. Prickly heat

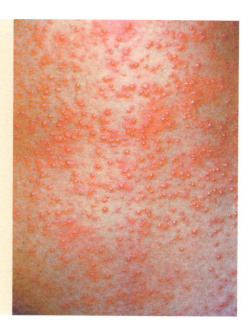

Prickly heat develops when the narrow ducts carrying sweat to the skin surface get clogged. The trapped sweat causes inflammation, which produces irritation (prickling), itching, and a rash of very tiny blisters. It is most common in warm, humid climates. Prickly heat tends to occur on areas of the body where skin touches skin, such as under the breasts, on the inner thighs, and under the arms.

SUN-DAMAGED SKIN

Although sunshine is essential for health and vitamin D production in the skin, excessive exposure to sun's ultraviolet (UV) light can be extremely hazardous. Prolonged exposure to UV light may result in DNA damage that can be accounted for premature skin aging, wrinkling, and irregular pigmentation. Different types of skin cancer—including squamous cell carcinoma, basal cell carcinoma, and malignant melanoma—are linked to excessive sun exposure. Depending on its wavelength, UV light is classified into three categories: UVA, UVB, and UVC. It is believed that UVB is responsible for more of the damaging effects of UV light.

The amount of UV light reaching the earth's surface is proportional to the depletion of the protective property of the ozone layer that is composed of O3 molecules that block much of the UV light from reaching the surface of the earth. Excessive sunlight may cause various skin problems, including premature aging, loss of skin elasticity, development of wrinkles, dark circles around the eyes, and unattractive skin pigmentation. Spending time outdoors makes it difficult to avoid excessive exposure to the sunlight. In the ozone-depletion countries, this may also increase the risk of exposure to harmful sun radiation. UV light is more intense between 10:00 AM and 3:00 PM, in the summer, and at higher altitudes. The appearance of sun-damaged skin is well recognized from normal chronological aging. Avoiding prolonged exposure to sunlight and regular usage of sunblock lotions are strongly recommended by the dermatologists who are working to prevent skin cancer.

There are a number of products and treatments available to minimize some of the signs of sun damage. Sunblock products contain substances such as para-aminobenzoic acid (PABA) and benzophenone, which absorb UV light. PABA may irritate the skin or cause an allergic reaction in some people. PABA does not instantly attach to the skin to exert its function. Therefore, sunscreen products containing PABA or benzophenone must be used at least thirty minutes before exposure to the sun's radiation. Sunblocks containing zinc oxide or titanium dioxide constitute a thick physical barrier that prevents all sunlight from reaching to the skin and can be used on small, sensitive areas.

PROTECTION FROM UV RAYS

Unprotected skin that is exposed to the sun for a long period of time show more irregularity in color. Excess sunlight can turn freckles into brown sunspots and increase wrinkles and sagging, which gives a very aged look to the skin. It is now generally accepted that the risk of melanoma or skin cancer is significantly increased by sun exposure. When skin is exposed to UV light, it endures particular changes to protect against the harmful effects of UV light. For example, the epidermis thickens to partially block the UV light.

Figure 4.5. Sunburned skin

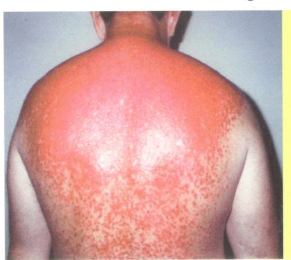

Sunburn is literally a burn on the skin due to UV radiation. The consequence of this burn is inflammation of the skin. Injury can start within thirty minutes of exposure.

The synthesis and accumulation of melanin is increased in melanocytes that, in turn, darken the skin color. This is a natural body defense in response to UV radiation since melanin protects the skin by absorbing the UV light and preventing the damaging of skin cells from deeper penetration into the skin. The quantity of melanin present in the skin is hereditary and depends on race and environmental factors—for example, the amount of daily sun exposure. Brief overexposure to ultraviolet light causes sunburn characterized by painful blushed skin, blisters and fever. Sunburn can be prevented by avoiding excessive sun exposure and by using sunscreens. People can get sunburned even on cloudy days because clouds do not filter ultraviolet light. Even sunscreens that are waterproof or water-resistant need to be reapplied after swimming.

Figure 4.6. Skin peeling on sunburned areas several days after the exposure

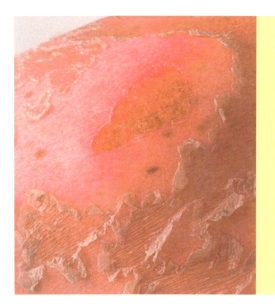

Sun exposure can cause first- and second-degree burns. It results when the amount of exposure to the sun or other ultraviolet light sources exceeds the ability of the body's protective pigment, melanin, to protect the skin. Sunburn in a very light-skinned person may occur in less than fifteen minutes of midday sun exposure.

Figure 4.7. Penetration of UV rays to the skin

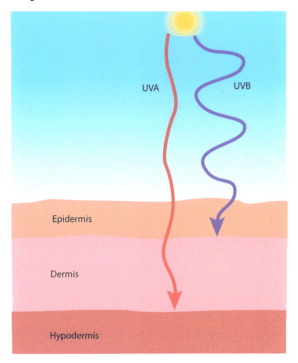

UVB, also known as tanning rays, has the strength to penetrate the epidermis that is composed of keratinocytes, basal cells, and melanocytes. UVB rays stimulate the melanocytes to produce more melanin, which is more commonly known as suntan. UVA penetrates through the epidermis and disperses in the dermis, the second major layer of the skin. UVA rays accelerate the aging process. Prolonged exposure to UVA damages collagen and elastin in the epidermis and reduces the size of this layer, allowing epidermis to start drooping and wrinkling.

DARK UNDEREYE CIRCLES

As people age, dark circles under the eyes, with shadows cast by puffy eyelids, may appear. Dark circles are characterized as round, uniform areas of pigmentation beneath each eye that affect both adult men and women. However, undereye circles can be observed in children as well. This tired and frustrated appearance can be embarrassing to some people, which may result in some degrees of social withdrawal. Although dark circles under eyes usually are not a sign of exhaustion or serious illness, they can make the individuals feel old and unhealthy.

Despite general belief, fatigue is not the main cause for undereye circles. Some of the most common causes of dark circles under eyes include heredity and lifestyle factors, such as smoking, alcohol consumption, and drinking caffeinated sodas. Other medical factors are allergies and nasal congestion, which dilates the veins and darkens the skin due to increased superficial blood flow. In addition, excess sun exposure results in pigmentation irregularities, particularly in people with higher level of skin melanin, and contributes to the development of dark undereye circles. Using sunblocks may reduce the appearance of the dark circles. Some reports indicate that thinning skin and the loss of fat and collagen that occurs in aged people make the reddish-blue blood vessels under the eyes more obvious. This can manifest as dark circles under the eyes.

Figure 4.8. Dark undereye circles

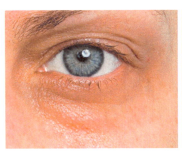 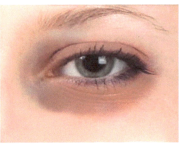

The skin around the eyes is some of the thinnest, most delicate skin of the entire body. The tiny blood vessels, or the capillaries, are much closer to the surface of the skin in this area. In people with persistent dark circles around the eyes, skin is not only thinner at this location but also more translucent. The combination of capillaries near the skin's surface and translucent skin makes this discoloration much more apparent.

AGING, SAGGING SKIN

Sagging and loose skin is usually a sign of aging; however, it can be seen even at a young age due to sudden weight loss. Although sagging is the hallmark of aging, in which the skin loses its elasticity, young individuals may experience it if adequate skin care is not taken (Figure 4.9). The onset of sagging skin can be delayed with proper skin care approach. Thus, an understanding of the major causes and knowledge about the preventive measures is inevitable in a well-planned skin care program.

ETIOLOGY OF SAGGING SKIN

As people age, the formation and deposition of collagen and elastin, two critical fibrous scleroproteins of the connective tissue and extracellular matrix, are decelerated dramatically. These two scleroproteins are responsible for maintaining the elasticity, firmness, and health structure of the skin. Thus, they help to prevent sagging and keep the skin firm against the gravitational pull. When the turnover of collagen and elastin starts to decrease, the skin becomes loose, saggy, and droopy due to the forces of gravity. This process is often accelerated by factors like overexposure to sunlight and free radicals. The main cause of skin sagging in younger population is caused by rapid weight loss (Figure 4.10). New mothers can also experience loose and sagging skin in the abdominal region after delivery. During pregnancy, the skin stretches substantially, while after the delivery abdominal volume loss results in it abrupt contracting, leading to skin sagging (Figure 4.11).

Figure 4.9, Aging, sagging skin

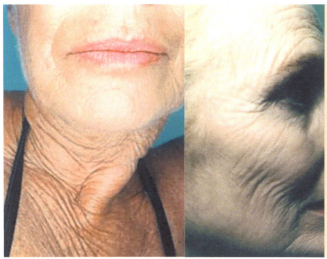

Four main causes leading to aging, sagging skin are free radical damage, decreased collagen production, decreased production of new skin cells, and low levels of hyaluronic acid

Figure 4.10. Sagging skin due to sudden weight loss

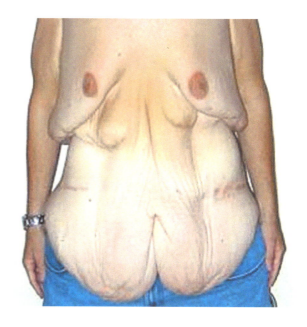

Loose and sagging skin develops especially in the upper arms, abdomen, and thighs, As the skin stretched due to accumulated fats, it is not given enough time to tighten itself. It is a common sign that manifests in obese people after losing too much weight rapidly.

NATURAL SKIN AGING

The aging of skin is a process that is comprised of gradual loss of tone and thickness, development of age sunspots, and changes in vascular system. All these conditions lead to changes in the appearance of the skin, sagginess, folds, and wrinkles. These unwanted consequences of skin-aging have developed a branch of scientific skin care known as skin rejuvenation. People who have wished to prevent the signs of aging have long sought facelifts and body contouring and other wrinkle-reducing procedures. However, it takes more than tightening loose skin to restore a youthful appearance. Skin aging appears to be also dependent on the factors like changes in facial bones that take place as people age, which contributes to an aged look.

There are two distinct cause of skin aging: first, aging caused by hereditary factors—called intrinsic (internal) aging—and, second, aging caused by environmental factors—known as extrinsic (external). A very common example of the later factor is prolonged exposure to the sun radiation. Unfortunately, aging by inheritance cannot be prevented; however, there are habits that make skin age faster and can be managed in order to substantially reduce the process of aging. Preventable environmental factors that intensify intrinsic aging include sun exposure and smoking.

Figure 4.11. Postpregnancy sagging skin in abdominal area

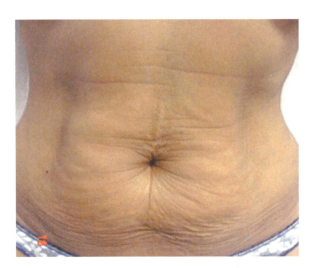

One of the most pronounced changes during pregnancy can result from stretched skin as the body shapes itself to hold the fetus for nine months. The skin of the breast and tummy is most often affected by hormonal changes and increased size during pregnancy.

Figure 4.12. Facial wrinkles associated with skin aging

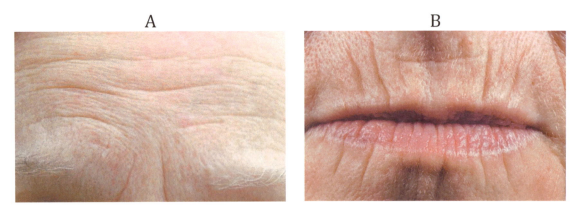

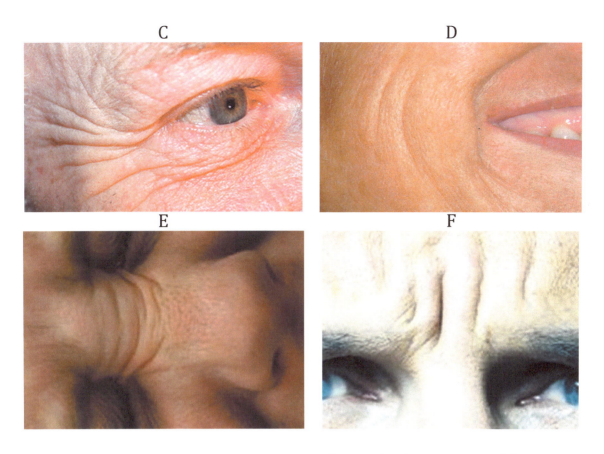

The most common facial wrinkles due to aging are forehead wrinkles (A), smokers' lines (B), crow's-feet wrinkles (C), laugh lines or nasolabial folds (D), bunny lines (E), and frown lines (F).

BIOLOGY OF SKIN AGING

At the cellular and molecular level, aging is associated with senescence and the truncation of telomeres. Telomeres are the terminal portions of chromosomes in each cell cycle. Telomere shortening ultimately results in cell-cycle arrest or programmed cell death once a critical length is reached. At the histological level, photoaging is manifested as flattening of the dermal-epidermal junction resulting in decreased nutrient transfer between the layers. In addition, chronic inflammation, elongated and collapsed fibroblasts, disorganized collagen fibrils with overall decrease in collagen levels, and the accumulation of elastin are accounted for the skin aging.

SMOKING AND SKIN AGING

It has been reported that smoking cigarettes or exposure to smoke by simply being a secondhand smoker significantly hastens the process of skin aging and increases skin wrinkles. The notion that exposure to cigarette smoke is as damaging to aging skin as exposure to the sun's ultraviolet rays has raised a great deal of concern. Cigarette smoke depletes vitamin C from the body, which is a key ingredient for collagen synthesis and collagen deposition in the connective tissue and extracellular matrix. Collagen is a fibrous protein that connects and supports other bodily tissues, such as skin, bone, tendons, muscles, and cartilage. Collagen makes up about 25% of the total amount of proteins in the body. It is generally referred as the glue that holds the body together. Thus, the appearance of skin wrinkling, especially facial wrinkles, has been attributed to the loss of collagen, which keeps the skin plump and curvy.

Figure 4.13. Smoking and skin aging

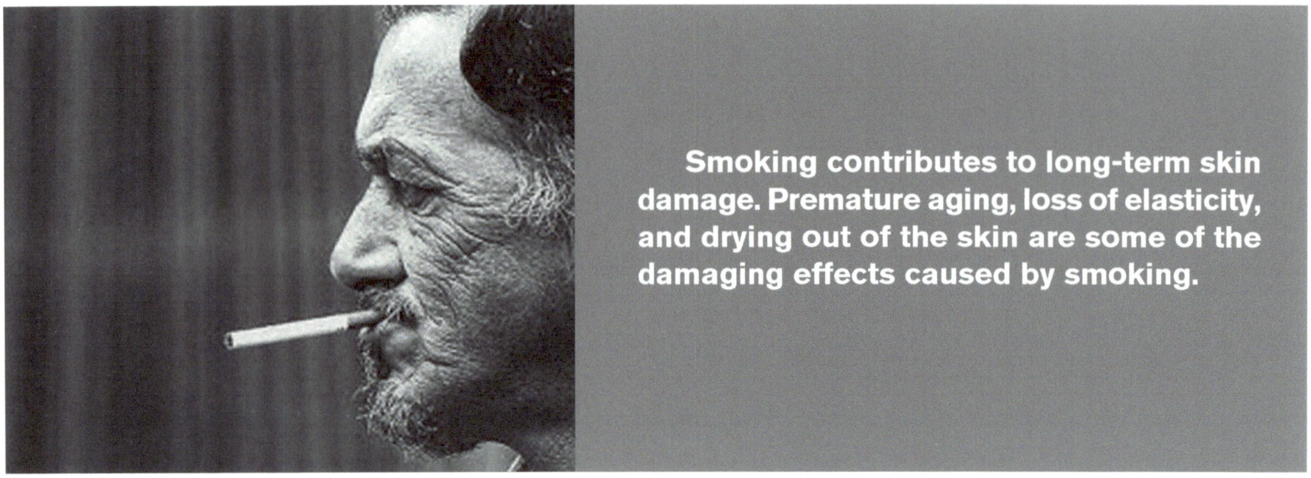

Smoking contributes to long-term skin damage. Premature aging, loss of elasticity, and drying out of the skin are some of the damaging effects caused by smoking.

LACK OF EXERCISE AND SKIN AGING

Exercise should inevitably be an important part of every antiaging skin care syllabus. Inactivity and reduced blood flow to muscles and skin considerably contributes to skin aging. Exercise prevents the weakness of the muscles, particularly the facial muscles, that keep the skin lifted up. Sedentary older adults are also at higher risk for dementia or cognitive and intellectual deterioration. The immune system is also strengthened through exercise. Most importantly, however, exercise delays the effects of skin aging by increasing the strength and tolerance of the skin to microbial infection.

REACTIVE OXYGEN SPECIES (ROS) AND SKIN AGING

Long-term introduction to UVA radiation accelerates intrinsic aging through the formation and detrimental effect of reactive oxygen species (ROS). ROS triggers signaling molecules and cellular pathways that lead to increased expression of inflammatory cytokines and the upregulation of collagenase. As the result, collagen breakdown is accelerated and leads to the loss of skin connective tissue volume and skin aging manifested by wrinkles and folds. UVB radiation can also contribute to this aging process by causing direct DNA mutations.

EXTREME HOT OR COLD WEATHER

Cold winds and low temperatures make skin dry and contribute to the conditions that promote aging of the skin. Using moisturizer can prevent skin dry if exposure to cold weather in inevitable. On the other hand, indoor environments with faulty heating system or places with hot, dry air for a long period of time may promote dry skin. Therefore, indoor administration of moisturizers is strongly recommended as heated rooms can be very drying to skin. Having a humidifier installed in homes with dry and hot central air-forced heaters help keep the skin more relaxed and reduces the risks contributing to the skin aging.

STRESS AND ALCOHOL CONSUMPTION

Stress and anxiety cause unnecessary facial expressions like frowning and eye wrinkles. Repetitive and prolonged facial expressions lead to permanent fine lines and wrinkles as well as conformation of muscles in the face to the facial expression.

As skin ages and loses its elasticity, the skin stops springing back to its line-free position and the grooves become permanently engraved on the face as fine lines and wrinkles. Some people use alcohol to reduce the level of their stress. However, alcohol has an adverse effect and promotes the aging of skin by dilating small blood vessels in the dermis and increasing blood flow near its surface. Over time, these blood vessels can become permanently damaged, creating a flushed appearance and broken vessels on the skin's surface.

STRETCH MARKS

Stretch marks (*striae*) are one of the most common and undesirable cosmetic defects of the skin. Stretch marks occur when skin is overstretched and its elasticity cannot prevent deformation to the skin matrix. Stretch marks can be found in different extents on the skin of all people. The extent of a stretch mark depends on health condition, lifestyle, occupation, or physical activities.

The most common occurrence of stretch marks is in women after pregnancy. During the pregnancy, the skin is pulled to accommodate the size of rapidly growing abdomen. In addition to pregnancy, rapid growth at puberty during a growth spurt or during weight gain may result in stretch marks. Except the face and neck, the abdominal area, hips, thighs, arms, breasts, and shoulders are the most commonly affected sites. Stretch marks usually are pale, but many women may develop purple stretch marks after pregnancy. The color will eventually fade out with time, but in most cases, the marks will stay (Figure 4.14).

Figure 4.14. Stretch marks in the abdominal area

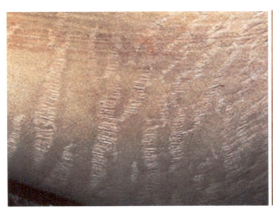 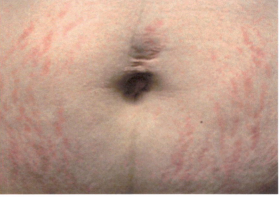

Stretch marks occur on the body when skin is stretched and torn. The torn skin is replaced by scar tissue. This usually occurs as a result of rapid growth such as in puberty, pregnancy, or muscle building. It is possible to remove stretch marks using laser surgery.

TREATMENT OF STRETCH MARKS

Although there are many creams and lotions available, there are none to effectively remove stretch marks. Using special oil formulas available in the market that increases flexibility of the skin may have some minimal effect in reducing the appearance of the stretch marks during pregnancy. Stretch marks can be removed considerably by laser resurfacing but cannot be totally diminished as yet. Skin tightening and photodynamic skin rejuvenation can be further utilized as cosmetic procedures to treat stretch marks. Microdermabrasion or laser therapy for collagen remodeling may also be useful to make the stretch marks look slightly better and less visible. It is suggested that skin tightening using the Thermage technique may reduce stretch marks by a greater extent.

SCAR FORMATION

In the skin, abnormalities in the wound-healing process may lead to delayed healing or excess fibrosis and scar formation. Scars are fibrous tissues that replace normal tissue at the site of injury. When scarring occurs in skin, it may result in significant cosmetic, functional, and psychological impairments. Minor scars are usually flat and pale, with a trace of the original wound. Compared to other type of scars, they contain less collagen and connective tissue cells. In contrast, overhealing results in excessive collagen deposition and the formation of keloids or hypertrophic scars. They are characterized by excess amounts of thick unorganized collagen fibers that are randomly aligned as compared to the normal basket-weave orientation in unwounded tissue.

Hypertrophic scars are red, raised, and itchy lumps on the skin and are limited to the boundaries of the original wound. Hypertrophic scars represent the dermal equivalent of fibroproliferative disorders that occur after injuries involving the deep dermis, while superficial wounds to the skin heal with minimal or no scarring. Keloids that occur in about 10% of population are larger and grow beyond the original wound zone. Analysis of scar-inducing factors has been the center of attention in many studies. Excess activity of growth factors released from platelets and inflammatory cells in the first phase of wound healing, failure to eliminate collagen-producing cells (myofibroblasts) from wound granulation tissue, and reduced collagen breakdown at later time points have been considered as conditions that lead to the formation of hypertrophic scars.

Furthermore, increased inflammatory responses resulting in excess release of cytokines and fibrotic growth factors have been shown to promote keloid and hypertrophic scar formation. More than 70% of burn wounds, traumatic injuries, or postsurgical procedures in skin develop hypertrophic scars that can result in tissue disfigurement or the disruption of normal organ function. Better understanding of differences in cellular and molecular mechanisms involved in normal skin wound healing and development of hypertrophic scars may provide valuable information that can be used to prevent scar formation.

Figure 4.15. Scar formation

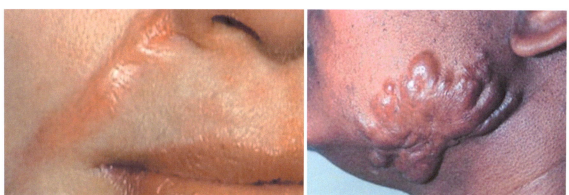

Wound healing is the complex and dynamic mechanism that results in the restitution of damaged skin. The process of wound healing is comprised of a continuous process of repair in which different cells—such as platelets, fibroblasts, epithelial cells, endothelial cells, and inflammatory cells—interact with extracellular matrix molecules, growth factors, and cytokines. Aberrations in this process may result in chronic nonhealing wounds or the deposition of excess collagen and scar formation. Abnormal overproduction of collagen at the site of injury results in hypertrophic (A) or keloid (B) scars.

CELLULITES

The term *cellulite* refers to the dimpled appearance of the skin that appears on hips, thighs, and buttocks. The lumpiness of cellulite is caused by fat deposits that push and distort the connective tissues beneath skin, leading to the characteristic changes in the appearance of the skin. Cellulite is not related to the condition known as cellulitis, which is a spreading bacterial infection of the skin and tissues beneath the skin. Cellulite develops in the subcutaneous fat layers and gives the skin a dimpled or orange peel–like appearance (Figure 4.16). This layer of fat is structured into specific chambers surrounded by fibrous tissue implanting pressure on the underlying fat. As the result, skin affected by cellulite becomes wavy and shows irregular or regular bumps and depressions. This condition can be very obvious once one tightens the buttocks or thigh muscles, the pelvic regions, lower limbs, and abdomen.

Surprisingly, 90% of postadolescent women develop cellulite at some time during their life much more often than men. The causes of cellulite are inadequately understood. Hormones play a crucial role in the formation of cellulite. For example, the female sex hormone estrogen, has been suggested for principally setting off and intensifying the cellulite. Other factors such as genetic, gender, race, diet, and distribution of subcutaneous fat play important roles in the susceptibility of an individual to cellulite. In addition, an elevated-stress lifestyle may cause an increased level of so-called fight-or-flight hormones, catecholamines, released in response to stress, which have also been linked to the development of underlying fat tissue and cellulite.

Figure 4.16. Cellulite

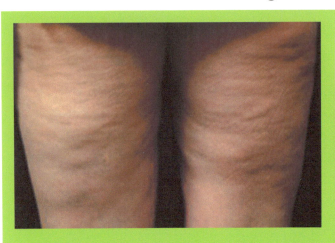
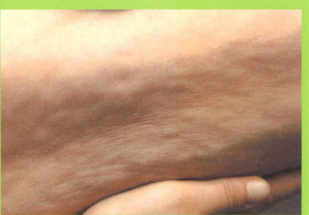

Cellulite is a modification of skin topography evident by skin dimpling and nodularity caused by the herniation of subcutaneous fat within fibrous connective tissue, leading to a padded or orange peel–like appearance.

TREATMENT OF CELLULITES

Topical lotions that contain antioxidants and anti-inflammatory ingredients are thought to be effective for cellulite reduction as they encourage the blood flow. There are also creams available that contain herbs, minerals, and vitamins to help skin become softer and smoother. Other technically advanced treatments available for cellulite treatment include laser therapy, ultrasound, suctioning devices, or electromagnetic impulses. Thermage has also been suggested for reducing cellulite. One effective and practically sound procedure for minimizing cellulite is mesotherapy, which will be discussed thoroughly in later chapters.

Briefly, mesotherapy involves delivering a fat-dissolving drug directly into the areas affected by cellulite, making it better by gradually breaking down the subcutaneous accumulated fat. Hyaluronidase is an enzyme that's very effective in the treatment of cellulite as it digests the links of fibrous tissues formed between the lobules of fat. Collagenase, an enzyme that degrades collagen, can be administered along with mesotherapy. It helps in the disintegration of fibrous bands that are binding to the lobules of fat.

Partial or ineffective treatment may only shrink fat lobules by causing a loss of water from the fat cells. Upon rehydration of fat cells overtime, signs of cellulite will reappear. Many women leave the cellulite untreated after they have been financially and emotionally exhausted.

PIGMENTATION DISORDERS (VITILIGO)

The amount of pigment in the skin is determined by the amount of melanin being produced by the skin cells called Melanocytes. Loss of pigment (hypopigmentation) can be caused by the lack of melanocytes that synthesize skin pigments (melanin), malfunctioning of melanocytes, exposure to cold chemicals, or certain infections. Vitiligo is an example of hypopigmentation. Increased skin melanin or hyperpigmentation may be caused by skin irritation, hormonal changes, aging, a metabolic disorder, or sun damage. Melasma, freckles, and age spots are examples of hyperpigmentation.

Figure 4.17: Hypopigmentation

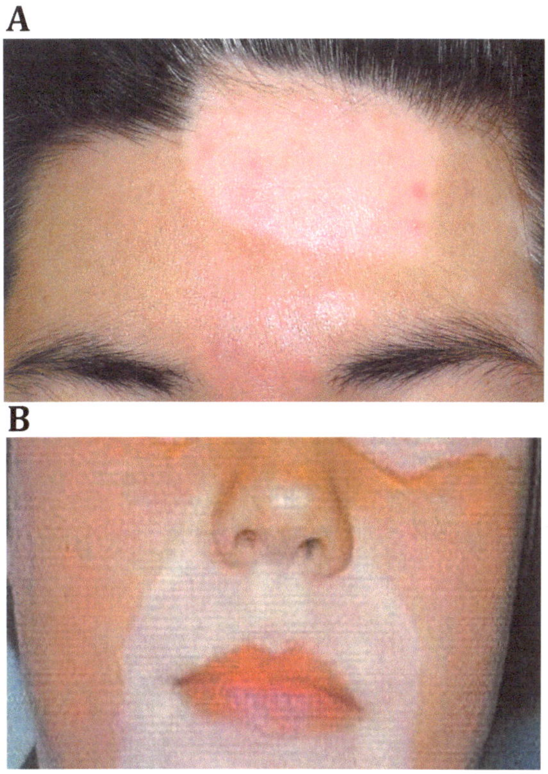

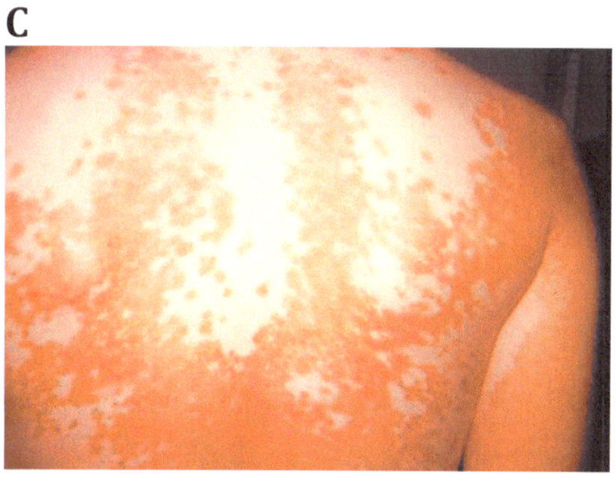

Vitiligo is a pigmentation disorder in which melanocytes in the skin are destroyed or are unable to function. It is characterized by the appearance of depigmented patches, more commonly on sun-exposed areas of the body such as on the face (A-B) or back (C).

HYPERPIGMENTATION

Undesired changes in skin pigmentation are a major concern to many women and men. The darker spots arise from a disorder of specialized skin cells, melanocytes, responsible for the production of skin pigment. Hormonal stimulation, oral birth control pills, sun exposure, or taking some prescribed or over-the-counter drugs that cause photosensitivity (like tetracycline antibiotics used to treat acne) are believed to be cause formation of darker skin spots, and generally described as hyperpigmentation. Some of the alterations in the skin pigmentation are hereditary, and some are due to hormonal changes like melasma (mask of pregnancy). Pigmented skin can be seen as age spots, liver-brown pigmentation, freckles, sunburns, and posttraumatic pigmentation. The darker spots on the facial skin or neck are difficult to treat.

Treatment of skin hyperpigmentation is not easy, and the results can often be much less than expected. These circumstances often cause a lot of anxiety among people seeking solutions to their skin with dark patches. Treatment of hyperpigmentation must be initiated by informing the patients to avoid sun exposure and applying sunblocks effectively by the efficient covering of sun-exposed body areas. Lightening topical products ranging from a cucumber extract to creams with vitamin C or hydroquinone have been suggested for the treatment and care of hyperpigmentation. However, it is not clear how they are as effective as avoiding sun radiation.

Chemical peels and microdermabrasion may reduce dark skin patches and melasma to a large extent. Further reduction of hyperpigmentation can be achieved by a chemical peel called Cosmelan that blocks melanocytes and literally prevents skin darkening for extended periods of time. Cosmelan is usually available in the medical spas and laser clinics, and its application includes performing a peel by a skin care therapist. The client must continue using Cosmelan cream at home for several months following treatment in the clinic.

Figure 4.18. Hyperpigmentation

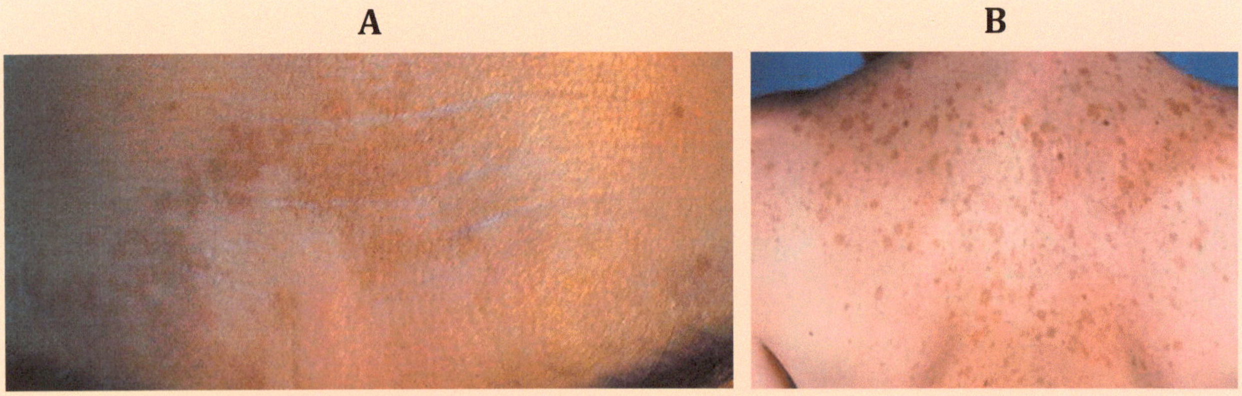

Hyperpigmentation is caused by an excess production of melanin associated with a number of conditions particularly excess sun exposure. (A) Face; (B) back.

MELASMA AND CHOLASMA

Melasma is a widespread skin pigmentation that appears as blotchy, tanned, or gray-brown areas on the face. It develops slowly and fades overtime. The pigmentation is due to the overproduction of melanin by the melanocytes. The most common areas of melasma onset are, bridge of nose, brow, cheeks, chin, and upper lip, as well as forearms and neck. Females show the sign of melasma more often than men. Compared to women, the frequency of melasma in men is as little as 5–10%.

Dark-skinned individuals that have more active melanocytes than those with light skin produce more pigment, which increases when stimulated. The causes of melasma still warrant considerable investigation; however, consumption of birth control pills, heredity, pregnancy, cosmetics, hormone therapy, drugs that make the skin more susceptible to light damage, and sun exposure often results in the development of melasma. Melasma associated with pregnancy, also known as chloasma or the mask of pregnancy, often fades a few months after delivery.

Melasma is categorized into epidermal, dermal, and mixed types. Epidermal melasma appears as a well-defined border of dark brown color and is more obvious under black light. Dermal melasma shows poorly defined borders. The response of dermal melasma to treatment is not as good as the epidermal type. Mixed-type melasma often appears as a combination of both light and brown pigmentations, which partially improve with treatment.

Figure 4.19: Melasma

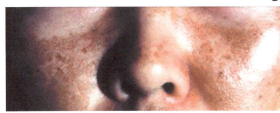

Melasma is common in women, especially pregnant women, and those who are taking oral or patch contraceptives. Melasma associated with pregnancy is also known as chloasma or the mask of pregnancy.

TREATMENT OF MELASMA

A range of topical creams that contain hydroquinone is available for the treatment of melasma. Hydroquinone is a commonly used skin-lightening ingredient in topical lotions. In addition, creams containing tretinoin, corticosteroids, glycolic acid, or azelaic acid—which may be combined with hydroquinone to enhance the skin-lightening effect—are also used for the treatment of melasma. Laser therapy, microdermabrasion, and/or chemical peels have also been used and proven to reduce signs of melasma. In addition to medication and procedures applied for the treatment of melasma, using sunscreens appears to be essential for blocking the UV radiation and preventing of the skin hyperpigmentation. Sun exposure can trigger melasma because the pigment-producing cells in the skin or melanocytes are stimulated by the UV light from the sun.

MOLES

Moles and brown spots are common in all individuals, especially people with light skin. The average number of moles in an individual can range from a few to over a hundred. The most important concern about moles is that skin cancer or melanoma can develop in or near a mole. People with larger moles should have their skin examined by a dermatologist on a regular basis. Moles appear in different shapes, sizes, and colors. They can be flat or raised with or without hair and may be brown, pink, black, or blue in color. If a mole becomes irritated, unpleasant in appearance, or if skin cancer is a concern, it can be removed by a qualified physician or plastic surgeon.

Usually, the procedure known as surgical excision involves local anesthesia, cutting out the mole, and stitching the skin closed. Moles can also be removed using a surgical blade to shave it away. This method must be performed by a surgeon in clinic to prevent skin disfigurement or infection. It is reported that sun exposure may increase the number of moles; therefore, protection form sunlight may be the first measure taken to reduce the chance of skin cancer associated with moles.

Applying sunscreen and protective clothing and avoiding tanning beds are highly advised. All types of moles need to be carefully examined before their removal. Often, it may require a removal of a small portion of the mole to make sure that it is not cancerous or precancerous. As an alternative to surgical excision, moles can be erased by photodynamic therapy and/or laser procedure. Removal of moles on medical grounds when there is a suspicion that a mole may develop into cancerous or precancerous states is usually covered by local medical insurance and a health care plan. Various brown or light brown spots on the skin can be successfully treated with satisfactory cosmetic means. As there are many types of such lesions, the first step is to have them correctly diagnosed and assessed.

Figure 4.20. Moles

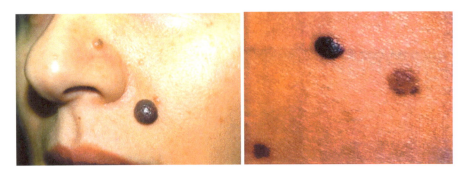

Moles occur when melanocytes grow in cluster instead of being spread throughout the skin. Most moles are not cancerous, but they may pose cosmetic skin problems.

ROSACEA

Rosacea is a chronic skin condition described by facial inflammation, tenderness, blushing, and erythema. Rosacea can affect a wide spectrum of people with different genetic and ethnic backgrounds and skin types, but it is most commonly seen in Caucasians—especially those who have lighter skin, blonde hair and blue eyes—and those who go red in the face easily. The exact cause or the age of rosacea onset is not clear; however, it is more frequently seen in adults between thirty and fifty years of age. Heredity and environmental factors are believed to play a role in the development of rosacea.

Initially, the redness may appear periodically, but over time, it becomes more pronounced and persistent. If not treated, it may appear as bumps and pimples. General symptoms include a puffy nose and visible blood vessels in the center of the face that can ultimately progress to the cheeks, forehead, chin, and nose. Eyes may become inflamed, red, and runny. The condition can be aggravated by the excessive use of alcohol, hot drinks, certain foods, stress, and exercise.

ROSACEA SUBTYPES

Rosacea occurs in four main subtypes known as papulopustular, phymatous, erythematotelangiectatic, and ocular. Erythematotelangiectatic rosacea is characterized with redness, flushing, and visible blood vessels. Patients with this subtype have a particularly very sensitive skin. Any medication applied to the face may cause intense irritation. Treatment may begin with topical sunscreen and/or an emollient cream, followed by topical lotions such as azelaic acid, metronidazole, or retinoid that reduce inflammation.

Papulopustular rosacea is often associated with bumps and pus-filled lesions that can be treated initially with topical antibiotics, including clindamycin or erythromycin, in combination with other topical medication containing azelaic acid, retinoid benzoyl, peroxide, sulfacetamide, or sulfur lotions.

Ocular rosacea involves eyes in which severe irritation redness, sensitivity, and watery condition are the main symptoms. If left untreated, ocular rosacea can impair the eyesight. Unfortunately, the treatment is limited to an eyelid hygiene regimen and the use of airdrops and antibiotics. Using intense pulsed light technology that introduces heat from light beams, coagulation of blood occurs within the dilated blood vessels, causing necrosis and the elimination of the blood capillaries responsible for the redness. Some bigger blood vessels may turn slightly gray before fading permanently. Visible results even after their first treatment can be satisfactory, but a series of at least three to five treatments are recommended to completely treat the symptoms.

Phymatous rosacea causes skin thickening and roughness, which can be treated by laser therapy, dermabrasion, or electrocautery. In the latter, thickened skin is removed by hot tip of an electrode.

Figure 4.21. Subtypes of rosacea

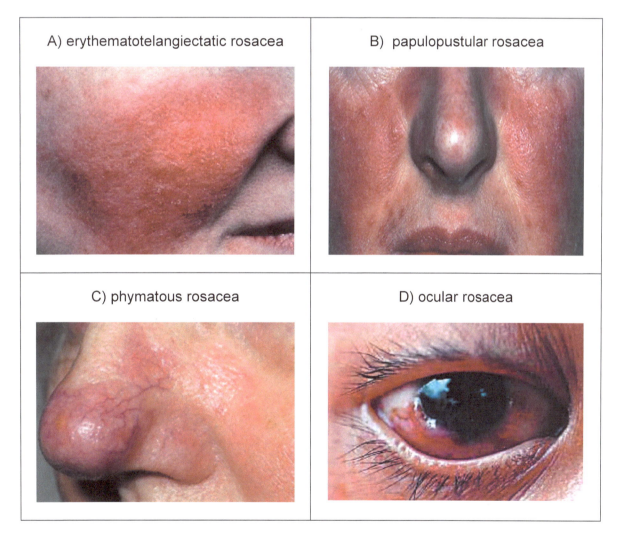

ACNE VULGARIS

Acne is a term used for an eruptive disease of the skin. It caused by an imbalance of skin-oil production and its depletion. Generally, overproduction or accumulation of skin oil (sebum) and associated inflammatory changes and infection are considered as the major etiology for acne. Acne is one of the most common of all skin problems that affect almost all age groups. However, acne generally begins during adolescence, and teenagers are more prone to developing acne. It is estimated that as many as 80% of people between twelve and twenty-five years of age suffer from acne, causing embarrassment, anxiety, and social retreat.

Acne mostly develops on the face, but common areas of the skin where acne also appears are on the neck, back, chest, and shoulders. Severity of acne depends on skin condition, inheritance, skin care, lifestyle, and bacterial infection. Acne has been linked to hormonal changes during puberty that lead to the development and maturation of sexual features, but not with sexual activity.

CAUSES OF ACNE

The sebaceous glands secrete an oily substance called sebum, which empties onto the skin's surface through hair follicles. The cells shed more rapidly and stick together, plugging the opening of the hair follicle and resulting in whiteheads. When whiteheads are exposed to air, they form blackheads. Also, the mixture of oil and cells contributes to the bacterial infection. Noninflammatory acne occurs when sebum accumulates in form of white specks best known as whiteheads. The retention of dark particles (keratin formed by skin turnover) leads to the formation of blackheads. Inflammatory changes result in formation of pink or red pimples. The most common bacterial infection in acne is caused by the *Propionicum acnes*.

TYPES AND STAGES OF ACNE

Acne is developed in three main forms known as the comedones, papules/pustules, and nodules or mild, moderate, or severe stages, respectively. Comedones refer to early acne spots caused by blocked pores, with no redness and inflammation. Closed comedones are whiteheads, and open comedones are blackspecks or blackheads. At this stage, acne is considered as mild. During the development of moderate acne, when the early spots get larger and inflamed, they turn into papules and pustules. In severe acne, very large and deep swellings called nodules and cysts that may be painful can also develop. The increased pressure within the clogged follicle causes the wall of the follicle to rupture. As a result, sebum, bacteria, and shed skin cells escape into the surrounding tissue, forming papules, pustules, and nodules that can be large and painful. Nodules are localized accumulations of pus and skin oils and are infested with bacteria. They can be very tender to the touch.

Figure 4.22. Causes of acne

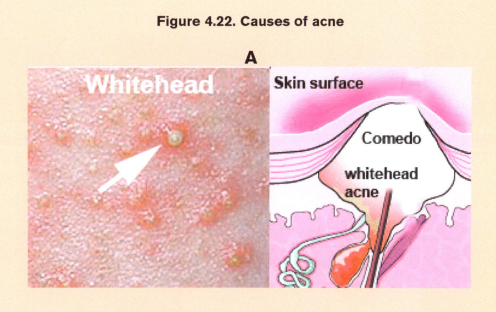

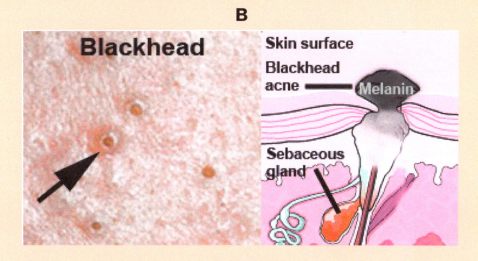

(A) Whiteheads result when a pore is completely blocked, trapping sebum, bacteria, and dead skin cells and causing a white appearance on the surface.

(B) Blackheads result when a pore is only partially blocked, allowing some of the trapped sebum, bacteria, and dead skin cells to slowly drain to the surface. The black color is due to the skin's own pigment, melanin, reacting with the oxygen in the air.

Ultimately, when nodules and cysts heal, acne scars will develop at the location, which may result in unpleasant look. Fortunately, these scars can be effectively treated with new medical aesthetic techniques and procedures. While in most people acne clears up after few years, many suffer from permanent scarring of the skin. Even when there are few physical marks left, the emotional ones can be devastating.

Figure 4.23. Types of Acne

A: Whiteheads

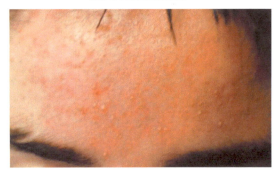

B: Blackheads

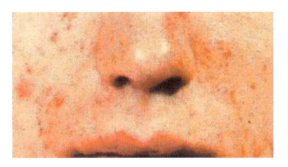

C: Papules

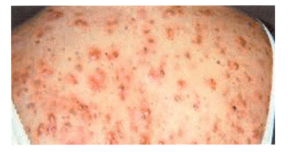

D: Pustules

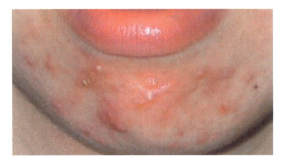

Acne vulgaris is one of the common types of acne among different people. It comes with different kinds of lesion like blackheads, whiteheads, papules, pustules, nodules, and cysts.

TREATMENT OF ACNE

People with chronic acne should seek medical treatment. Excessive overcleansing and scrubbing of the skin can dry out and irritate the skin, boost inflammation, and worsen the condition. Two main strategies for acne control are topical and systemic treatments. Patients should consult with a dermatologist to find out the exact type of their acne and to set goals and protocols for their treatment. Early management can substantially minimize the severity of acne and may reduce acne scarring. However, treatment may be necessary to carry out over months or often years. Methods for the treatment of acne depend on the severity of the condition, effectiveness of the method, side effects, gender, and personal preferences. Strategies for an effective treatment paradigm must be able to control the flow of sebum production, prevent new acne formation, remove dead skin cells, reduce the oiliness of the skin while preventing dryness, minimize bacterial infection of pores, and—finally—soothe and heal irritated skin.

The link between nutrition or certain diets and the abruption of acne is poorly understood. However, some people are allergic to certain foods that can make acne aggravated. A simple dietary modification, like limiting the consumption of excessively oily food, is beneficial and may help to prevent the aggravation of acne. Although there is little systemic information about the role of diet in acne control, improvements in the treatment of acne have been reported after less ingestion of chocolate or fatty fast foods. Therefore, in order to implement a successful treatment paradigm, a combination of therapy and management must be applied.

ACNE MEDICATION

Drugs that usually are used to treat mild acne are topical creams or lotions. They work by their antibacterial properties leading to the drying up or unclogging of the pores. The most commonly prescribed antibacterial drugs against acne are clindamycin, erythromycin, or Minocin. If topical antibacterials fail, other topical prescription drugs that help unclog the pores can be used. Most acne cleansers contain salicylic acid or benzoyl peroxide. Many companies sell over-the-counter products for acne such as topical retinoids, including Retin-A, Differin, or Tazorac. Isotretinoin is very effective, but is irritating to the skin and makes it more sensitive to sunlight.

Depending on the severity of the acne, some dermatologists prescribe systemic treatment by orally taken antibiotics including tetracycline, doxycycline, minocycline, or erythromycin. Acne patients should avoid taking oral antibiotics if the physician advises that they do not need one. For the most severe acne, when antibiotics are not effective, oral isotretinoin is considered as an effective treatment. Isotretinoin or Accutane is a vitamin A derivative, belonging to a class of medications called retinoids. Retinoids are usually used to treat skin problems. However, isotretinoin can have very serious side effects.

Therefore, isotretinoin is used to treat severe types of acne where other medications with less potential side effects have failed to improve the acne symptoms. Isotretinoin can be detrimental for a developing fetus. Due to pronounced side effects, Accutane is not recommended for mild to moderate acne. While it is true that many creams, oils, and greases can intensify the acne, there are many cosmetic products, including sunscreens and moisturizers, that do not affect acne and are usually labeled nonacnegenic or noncomedogenic. Oral contraceptives alleviate severe acne in women when their acne is aggravated during menstrual period. However, the effect can only be seen in two to four months. In some cases, large, inflamed nodules or abscesses can be treated by direct injections of corticosteroids into the acne.

TECHNIQUES FOR ACNE CONTROL

Many techniques can be applied alone or in combination in medical skin care clinics to alleviate the acne symptoms. For example, exfoliations of skin by microdermabrasion, chemical peels and/or photodynamic therapy (PDT) have been found to be highly effective. Direct elimination of bacteria in the skin using BLU-U and PDT along with evacuation of whiteheads by extraction of their content during these procedures has yielded to satisfactory results. Skin redness from acne can be treated with intense pulsed light (IPL). In chemical peels, glycolic acid is smoothed onto the skin for a short period of time to improve the appearance of cystic acne. Thermage treatment also may help skin tightening for the shrinking of sebaceous glands and the reduction of acne symptoms. Hormonal therapy is also an effective means to control acne abruption. Reduction of acne cysts may be achieved by microinjections of drugs such as steroids and/or antibiotics into cysts. Ingrown hairs can worsen acne. Laser hair removal can be performed prior to acne control to limit this problem.

DIET AND ACNE PROGRESSION

The necessity for a successful treatment that prevents problems associated with existing acne drugs motivated nutritionists to search for nutritional supplements that internally affect the progress of acne. There has been promising data on the use of certain minerals, together with vitamins, that influence acne improvement. While nourishing the skin, nutritional supplements can decrease inflammation and infections. Consumption of fresh fruits and vegetables as well as taking multivitamin supplements can make a difference. Vitamin A, in conjunction with vitamin E and zinc, has been shown to reduce sebum production and the buildup of keratin in the follicle. Regardless of the amount that is supplemented into the diet, vitamin E deficiency decreases the acceptable level of vitamin A in the human body.

Vitamin E is important for its interactions with selenium, which is an important antioxidant trace mineral. Selenium enhances the function of the enzyme glutathione perozidase. That plays an important role in preventing acne inflammation. Zinc is involved in the proper metabolism of the male sex hormone testosterone. Deficiency of zinc leads to an increase in the conversion of testosterone to dihydrotestosterone (DHT) hormone. It has been reported that DHT stimulates the production of sebum and keratin, which are primary factors in acne development.

AGGRAVATION OF ACNE

It is not scientifically evident whether certain foods or diets play a role in the progression of acne. Some eating habits may make acne worse. Eating too much fat such as deep-fried fast food, high-fat dairy products like cheese and ice cream, and refined carbohydrates and sugars are considered the worse types of food during an acne treatment program. Caffeine, which is abundant in coffee, tea, sodas, energy drinks, painkillers that contain caffeine, and chocolate usually stimulate the adrenalin glands and a subsequent release of stress hormones. Studies have linked stress to the abruption of acne and almost every other health condition.

Milk from pregnant cows contains hormones that are converted to DHT in skin glands, leading to sebum production and aggravation of acne. Mechanical tension such as scrubbing and squeezing could severely worsen acne and increases the risk of infection and scarring. Overcleansing by excess scrubbing or rubbing of the affected area causes irritation and skin dryness. Some cosmetics can promote acne by inducing acne to burst without causing blackheads. Sweating can intensify acne in some people, but sexual activity appears not to produce, cause, or aggravate it. Contraceptive pills and female sex hormone, progesterone, may exacerbate the condition. Some women tend to develop acne before their periods. Oil-free cosmetics are recommended for people suffering different degrees of acne. Noncomedogenic or nonacnegenic cosmetics are also available for use.

ACNE SCARS

Healed acne very often results in skin scarring. Acne scars varies in shapes and sizes. Most of the acne scars are irregular and have variable depth. The four main types of acne scars are the ice pick scar, the boxcar or angular scar, the rolling or round scars, and the hypertrophic scar (Figure 4.23 A–D). Ice pick scars, also called deep pits, are the most common and are a typical mark of acne scarring. Ice pick scars are narrow and sharp, which gives the skin a punctured appearance. They are usually narrower than 2 mm and extend into the deep dermis or subcutaneous layer. Unfortunately, ice pick scars are usually too deep to correct with skin resurfacing treatments such as microdermabrasion or laser resurfacing.

Boxcar or angular scars are similar to chicken pox scars and usually occur on the temple and cheeks. Boxcar scars may be shallow or deep with sharp vertical edges and are similar to the scars occurred by chicken pox. Rolling shallow scars are caused by damage under the surface of the skin and give the skin a wave-like appearance. They tend to be wide and shallow. Hypertrophic scars are itchy, red, raised, and generally confined within the boundary of the original wound. At the cellular level, they comprised of thick unorganized collagen bundle fibers and hypercellularity (increased number of myofibroblasts, endothelial cells, and blood vessels). Hypertrophic scars are often the result of severe acne lesions such as cysts or nodules.

Figure 4.23. Types of acne scars

(A) Ice pick scar

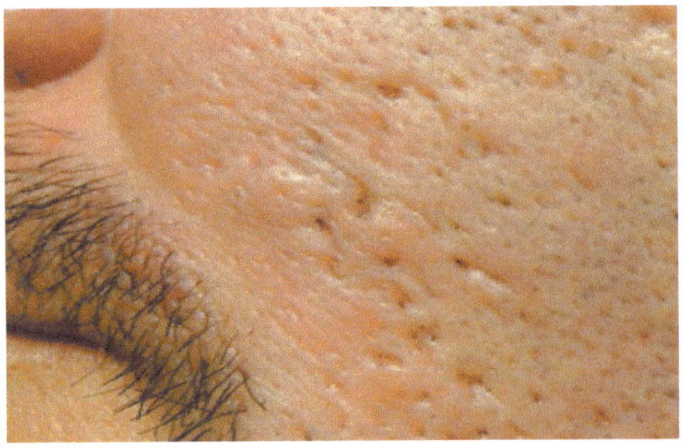

(B) Angular scar

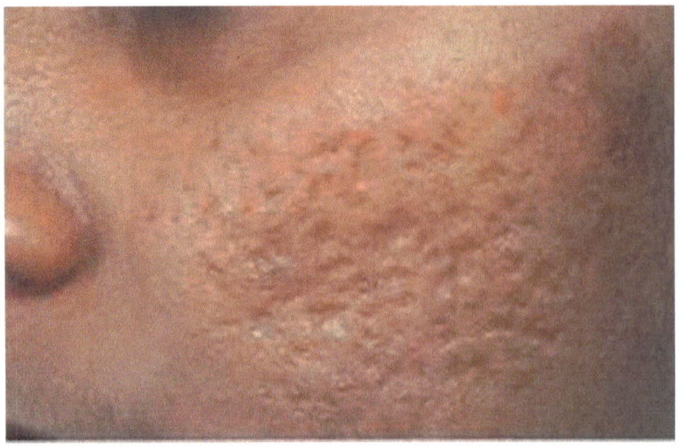

(C) Rolling or round scars

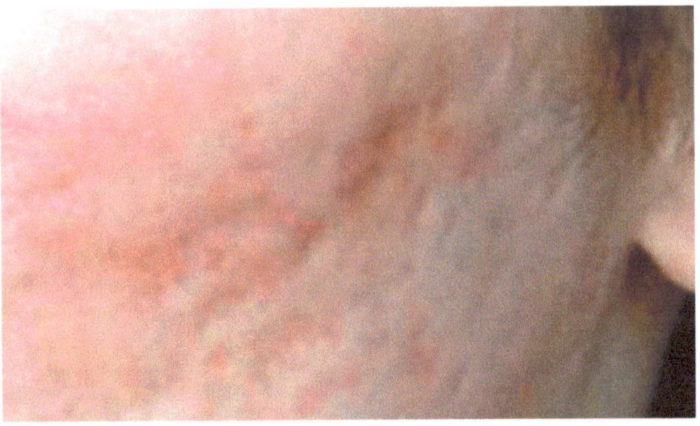

(D) Hypertrophic scar

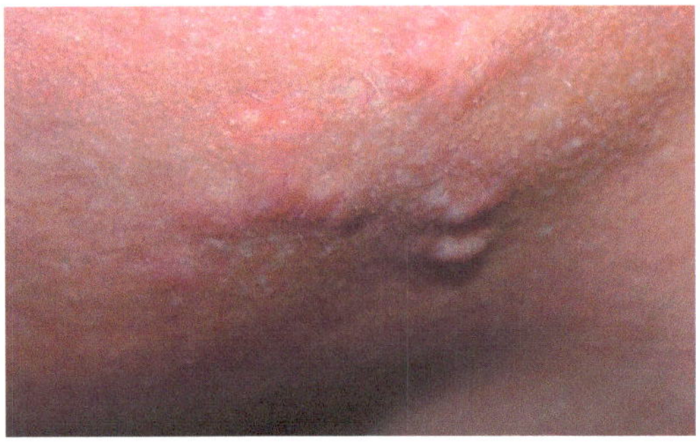

TREATMENT FOR ACNE SCARS

There are a number of available thrilling treatments for acne scars. Punch biopsy, microdermabrasion, PDT, and laser therapy can effectively treat acne scars. For ice-pick acne scars, a punch biopsy tool is used to make a surgical excision raging from 1.5 mm to 3.5 mm in diameters. The size of the tool is selected to match to the size of the scar. Under local anesthesia, the scar is excised and the skin edges are sutured together. The newly formed scar ultimately may not be obvious and are better suited to laser resurfacing techniques. Reduction of scar can be achieved by the removal of the outermost skin layer via microdermabrasion that uses a diamond tip to exfoliate the dead skin on the surface, deep chemical peels, or a laser micropeel.

Although temporary—lasting from three to six months—and effective only in shallow scars, the injection of filler hyaluronic acid into the depression of the scar in order to lift it flush to the surrounding skin is a popular method for resurfacing of the deep acne scars. Injection of steroid into the scar may also result in the softening of the scar and the improvement of the appearance of the skin. Light-based devices use the science of wavelengths of light to effectively treat red and brown scarring. Laser skin resurfacing is likely one of the best procedures to improve the appearance of atrophic scars such as ice pick or boxcar types. Lasers use high levels of energy to burn away scar tissue and reduces the appearance of scarring. A topical anesthetic must be applied to the skin an hour prior to the procedure to help with any discomfort.

Figure 24: Punch biopsy

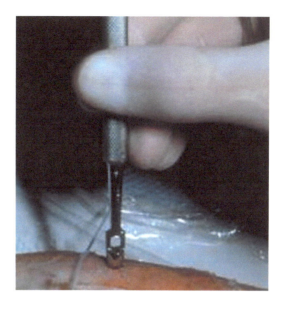

SPIDER VEINS

Telangiectasias or spider veins are small, thin, superficial capillaries that occur close to the surface of the skin. These dilated hair-sized small blood vessels usually are unattractively visible and may create social and psychological concerns for some people who are affected. Spider veins appear in red or bluish color with a linear, branch-like, or spider-shaped and dark center point. They can develop anywhere on the body, but they are mostly seen on the face around the nose, cheeks, and chin. They can also clearly appear on the legs, below the knee joint, and around the ankles.

Common symptoms include a burning or itching sensation. The cause of spider veins is not clear. They develop often as a result of localized and increased rate of angiogenesis or formation of blood vessels in an irregular pattern. Several factors including heredity, oral contraceptives, changes in the level of certain hormones, sun exposure, and natural aging process may also contribute to the development of spider veins. Other types of vein problems vary from small and large facial veins, to moderate and large varicose veins on the legs. Although unwanted blood vessels carry blood, the great majority of them, especially spider veins, are not functionally necessary and may be subjected to elimination.

Figure 4.25. Spider veins

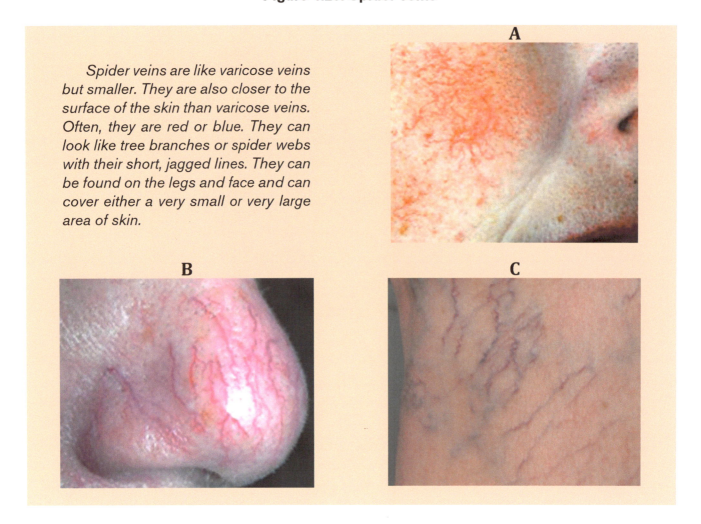

Spider veins are like varicose veins but smaller. They are also closer to the surface of the skin than varicose veins. Often, they are red or blue. They can look like tree branches or spider webs with their short, jagged lines. They can be found on the legs and face and can cover either a very small or very large area of skin.

SCLEROTHERAPY

Spider veins can be treated with sclerotherapy. It is a simple procedure whereby the visible veins are injected with a sclerosant, a substance that causes irritation of the veins' linings, leading to their subsequent destruction. Sclerotherapy is a proven, safe, effective, and virtually painless way of treating varicose and spider veins. It has been used, successfully, to treat both types of veins for over seventy-five years. In this procedure, hypertonic saline or sodium tetradecyl sulphate (Sotradecol) is injected while simultaneously monitoring the vein on an ultrasound screen. This allows for the accurate placement of the medication into the diseased veins that often leak and feed into the bulging surface veins. The medicine that is injected into the veins causes the vein walls to collapse. Polidocanol is also more commonly used in sclerotherapy.

Figure 4.26. Sclerotherapy

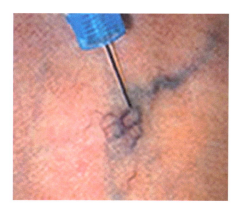

Image shows injection of a sclerosant into a patient's leg to treat varicose veins. The paths of the veins appear in purple/blue on the skin.

LASER TREATMENT FOR SPIDER VEINS

Removal of spider and small varicose veins by laser therapy is a nonsurgical approach for the treatment of unwanted superficial veins. Laser beams allow the delivery of a precise dosage of energy to each vein. A series of light pulses is delivered to the target without harming any surrounding tissues. The blood vessels planned for removal absorb the light energy and are gently heated in due course, which leads to a blood clotting within the vein. This, in turn, causes the blood vessel to collapse and be reabsorbed by the body as part of a natural healing process. Larger veins can be treated by injections.

ALOPECIA (HAIR LOSS)

The term alopecia refers to the loss of hair on the head or on any other part of the body. The most common reasons for hair loss are changes in hormone levels along with heredity and/or aging, stress, and some skin disorders. The type of hair loss can be diagnosed by examining the hair and skin. Hair loss that occurs on the head is generally called baldness. Hair loss is often of great concern to people for cosmetic reasons. Normally, in an average person, about a hundred scalp hairs fall out in a day. Hair loss in greater numbers per day may result in baldness.

The most common cause of hair loss is androgenetic alopecia. Dihydrotestosterone, male sex hormones, and testosterone—which are also present in females in small quantities—regulate hair growth. Testosterone stimulates hair growth in the pubic area and underarms. Dihydrotestosterone stimulates hair growth in the beard area while its excess release in the body causes hair loss at the scalp. Hair loss occurs in about 50% of men and to a lesser extent in women. Male-pattern hair loss begins at a young age. It appears as a losing of all the hair on the head top, but retains hair on the sides and back of the scalp.

In female-pattern hair loss the hairline typically stays intact, but hair loss begins on the top of the head and is usually a thinning of the hair rather than a complete loss of hair. Hair loss also results from drugs, especially chemotherapeutic agents seen in people battling with cancer. Infection of the skin with microbial agents (especially fungal infections), systemic illnesses, endocrine disorders, and nutritional deficiencies are other common causes of hair loss. Commercially available medications recommended for hair loss are known as minoxidil and finasteride. Other methods for the treatment of hair loss include hair transplantation, application of extensions, and corticosteroids.

Figure 4.27. (A–B) Male-pattern hair loss. (C–D) Female pattern hair loss.

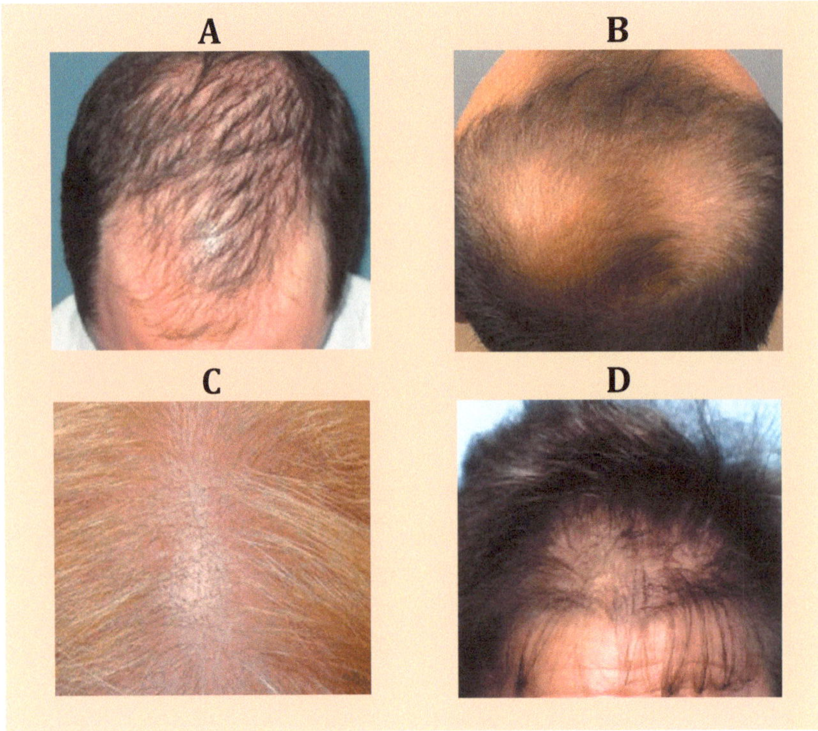

HIRSUTISM (EXCESSIVE FEMALE HAIR GROWTH)

The growth of coarse or dark hair in women in areas that are more usual of male hair patterns is called hirsutism. Hirsutism in women usually is seen in locations such as the mustache, beard, central chest, shoulders, lower abdomen, and back. Physiological or pathological overproduction of male hormones is considered the main reason for hirsutism. This condition in women may be accompanied by onset of acne, thickened vocals, and male-pattern hair loss. Treatment may include hormonal therapy and hair removal. Menstrual periods may become irregular or stop.

TREATMENT OF HIRSUTISM

Treatment for the excess hair itself is necessary if excess hair raises cosmetic issues. For excessive androgen, an oral contraceptive is used to reduce ovarian androgen production. Antiandrogenic drugs such as spironolactone, flutamide, and finasteride can also block the effects of testosterone, but may cause birth defects; therefore, they must be used together with oral contraceptives. Hair-removal strategies such as the application of topical hair-removal creams and/or laser therapy may be used to reduce the number of grown hair. Shaving does not increase the thickness of hair or the rate of hair growth and can be used as a temporary solution. Other common temporary hair-removal measures include plucking, waxing, and using a depilatory, which chemically removes hair at the skin surface. Electrolysis can give a more prolonged hair removal compared to other techniques.

Figure 4.28

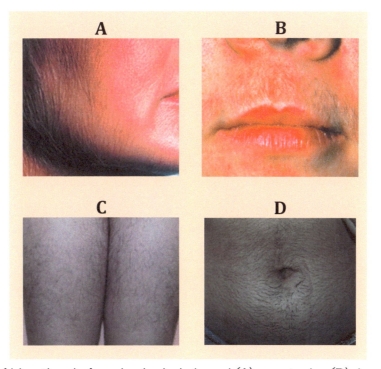

Common areas of hirsutism in females include beard (A), mustache (B), legs (C), and abdominal area (D)

PSEUDOFOLLICULITIS BARBAE (INGROWN BEARD HAIRS)

Pseudofolliculitis barbae, or ingrown beard hairs, refers to a condition when a tip of a curled hair grows backward and punctures the skin. This causes inflammation and a painful pimple. Pseudofolliculitis barbae can be diagnosed by its typical appearance and by teasing the tips of any ingrown hairs out of the skin with the point of a needle or sharp scalpel. The best preventive treatment is to stop shaving and grow the beard. If beard in not desired, the hair can be removed by depilatories, electrolysis, or with laser treatment. If shaving still is the only choice, the beard should be wet first and shaving should be in the same direction in which the hair grows.

Figure 4.29. Ingrown beard hair

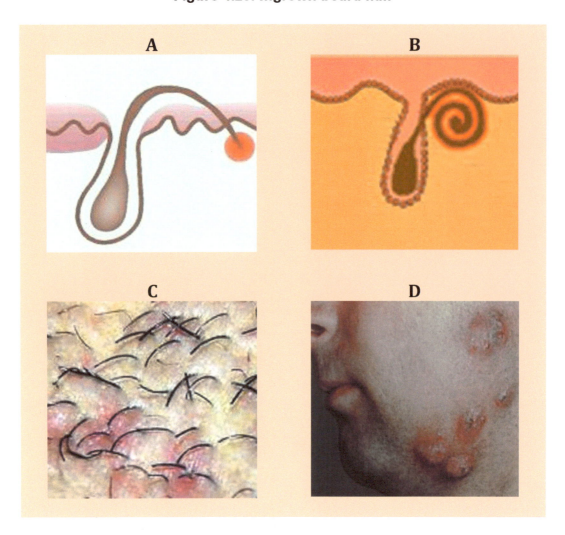

(A–B) Schematic illustration of ingrown beard hairs' etiology. (C) Thick bent hairs that grow backward into the skin. (D) Inflammations and pimples caused by ingrown beard hairs.

ADVANCED SKIN CARE STRATEGIES

Scientific research in the field of antiaging continues to give rise to new and promising treatment options. Each person has different skin conditions, as well as different expectations as to the results of proposed treatment. This is why there is a need for a very careful cosmetic consultation with a specialist and an experienced cosmetic physician or dermatologist for each client before undergoing any procedure. Antiaging goals can be accomplished by various nonsurgical and minimally invasive procedures, such as lasers and skin tightening. A number of treatments are available for improvement of aged skin as an alternative to the traditional skin tightening or facelifts; for example, botulinum toxin, radio-frequency treatment, laser resurfacing, laser collagen remodeling in conjugation with correction of volume loss by injectable cosmetic fillers, microdermabrasion, chemical peeling, and some topical treatments that will be discussed in detail in later chapters of this textbook. In addition, the following list comprises services that can be performed in a medical spa setting to improve the skin condition and should be part of skin rejuvenation program.

- antiaging treatment
- acne treatment
- acne scar treatment
- body toning
- breast toning
- cellulite reduction treatment
- drainage
- light therapy
- pale skin
- pigmentation
- rosacea treatment
- scar treatment
- stretch mark treatment
- rejuvenation
- impure skin
- face moisturization
- face toning
- wrinkles and fine lines

chapter 5

Microbiology for Medical Aestheticians

MICROBIAL SKIN INFECTION

INFECTION CONTROL IN SALONS AND SPAS

DISINFECTANTS

PREVENTION AND SAFETY MEASURES

SKIN PROTECTION IN FOOT SPAS

MYCOBACTERIUM FORTUITUM

COMMON MICROBIAL AGENTS IN SPAS AND SALONS

TREATMENT FOR BACTERIAL INFECTIONS

FUNGI INFECTIONS

CANDIDIASIS

NAIL FUNGUS

GREEN NAIL SYNDROME

TREATMENTS FOR NAIL FUNGUS

FINGERNAIL FUNGUS TREATMENT BY LASERS

INGROWN TOENAIL

RISKS OF ACRYLIC/ARTIFICIAL NAILS

CHAPTER 5

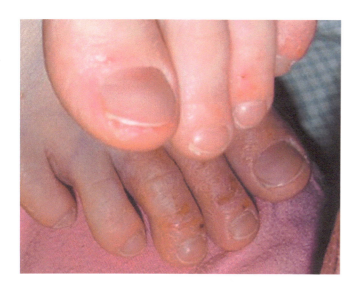

Microbiology for Medical Aestheticians

MICROBIAL SKIN INFECTION

Control of microbial infection is a real problem and a main concern for salons and spas. Beauty salons must, in fact, adopt and maintain the highest standards for dealing with infection control. The very first step is to understand which spores, viruses, and bacteria can be transmitted in a today's beauty salons and spas. Outbreaks of skin infections on the legs and feet of clients following spa pedicures have caused serious concerns about spa safety. Normally, unbroken and healthy skin provides an extraordinarily effective barrier against bacterial penetration and the onset of infections.

Although many bacteria come in contact with or are present on the skin as normal flora, they are unable to trigger an infection. Once the top protective layer of the skin is scratched, damaged, or traumatized with inflammation, it is more likely to be infected. Bacterial skin infections develop when bacteria enter the skin's surface through cuts, abrasions, allergic skin rashes, or other openings. Beauty salon clients with diabetes that have poor blood flow and weak immune systems are more prone to foot, finger, or skin infections. Other people at higher risk are those with human immunodeficiency virus (HIV) and cancer patients with a suppressed immune system due to medication and chemotherapy.

INFECTION CONTROL IN SALONS AND SPAS

The knowledge of dealing with clients with infection is necessary for medical aesthetic staff. It is important to decide what precautionary steps and safety measures are to be taken in order to keep the infection from spreading and/or transmitting to clients. The knowledge of providing consultation and for directing the clients to the physicians for cure is considered as one of the required skills for a medical aesthetics technician.

DISINFECTANTS

Professional use of approved and effective sterilization, disinfection, and sanitation solutions to minimize the risk of microbial infection has been a challenge for medical spa and salon management. Disinfectant for a salon and/or spa setting can be categorized into low-, intermediate-, and high-level grades. Low-level disinfectants are used primarily on surfaces to destroy some bacteria, viruses, and fungi. These include products such as quats (Ultracare, Barbicide, Zephiran, Faltrol Plus), phenols (Dettol, Lysol), and accelerated hydrogen peroxide (Accel AHP). Intermediate-level disinfectants eliminate most Mycobacterium (such as tuberculosis), most bacteria (such as pseudomonas and salmonella), viruses, and fungi. However, they are not effective against spores.

Intermediate-level disinfectants include products such as Accel AHP, alcohols (ethanol 70%, isopropanol) and halogens (bleach). High-level disinfectants kill effectively all mycobacterium, vegetative bacteria, viruses and fungi except for spores. Examples of high-level disinfectants are 2% glutaraldehyde, 7% Accel AHP (steam under pressure), dry heat, liquid and chemical sterilants such as virox's 7% accelerated hydrogen peroxide chemosterilant (Accel) and chemi-claves or chemical vapor. Glass bead, UV methods and boiling water are not considered as sterilization procedure.

PREVENTION AND SAFETY MEASURES

Practicing good hygiene and protecting the skin wounds from contamination can help prevent bacterial infections. Breaks in the skin, poor hygiene, and exposure to bacteria are risk factors for bacterial skin infections in a spa setting. There are primarily three routs of microbial transmission in today's salons and spas: (1) direct exposure (surfaces), (2) direct contact (skin to skin), and (3) vehicle-borne transmission (contaminated equipment and implements). Critical surfaces include items that penetrate the skin or mucous membranes, for example, needles and surgical instruments. The most appropriate method of control for this type of infection source is sterilization. Proper sterilization through autoclaving destroys almost all forms of microbial agents.

Figure 5.1

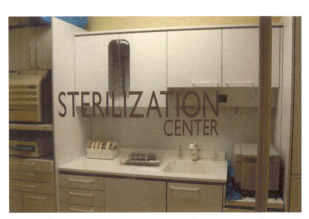

In eliminating contamination from outside sources, it is a good practice for an aesthetic clinic to install and use a high-tech self-contained sterilization center and water supply systems.

Semicritical surfaces include items that do not penetrate but come into contact with the skin or mucous membranes, like nippers. The most effective infection control strategy for this type of source is intermediate to high levels of disinfection, although sterilization could be used and would provide even greater infection control. Noncritical surface contact includes items that may come into contact with, but never penetrate, the skin or mucous membranes. Low levels of disinfection would be sufficient. In addition to establishing specific procedures for infection control, there are also a number of general common sense procedures that should always be followed. The highlights of these general and personal precautions are

(1) regular and frequent hand washing with soap, warm water, and/or alcohol-based products;
(2) wearing latex or vinyl gloves during procedures and changing the gloves when treating new clients;
(3) keeping sinks well stocked with antibacterial soaps and single service towels;
(4) working in well-ventilated rooms with smooth and nonporous surfaces, counters, and benches;
(5) keeping the equipment clean and in good working order and cleaning them prior to disinfection; and
(6) decontaminating the surfaces after every use and immediately disposing all contaminated waste using tightly sealed plastic bags.

SKIN PROTECTION IN FOOT SPAS

It is important to avoid using hair-removal creams, shaving, or waxing at least twenty-four hours before receiving treatment in a foot spa. Microorganisms in foot spas can enter through the skin, particularly broken skin caused by cuts and abrasions. Therefore, individuals with skin cuts should not come into contact with foot spa water. In addition, foot spa should not be used if skin has any open wounds, such as insect bites, bruises, and scratches. Initially, open wounds on the skin of feet and legs may not be noticeable, but they increase in size and severity over time and sometimes result in pus and scarring. Proper cleaning and disinfection can greatly reduce the risk of getting an infection by reducing the bacteria that can build up in the foot spa system.

Figure 5.2

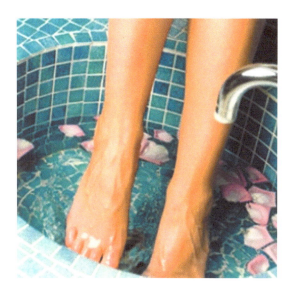

Foot care is as important as caring for any other part of the body. Taking a good footbath can help refresh the feet and take away the discomfort. However in public pools or foot spas, breaks in the skin, poor hygiene, and exposure to bacteria are risk factors for bacterial skin infections.

MYCOBACTERIUM FORTUITUM

Mycobacterium fortuitum, which can occur naturally in water and soil, is frequently reported to cause foot spa infections. The screens and tubes of foot spas often form dense layers of cells and proteins called biofilms, which can be very hard to remove. Biofilms are particularly good places for the bacteria to collect and grow. People who get treatments in foot spas must be aware of how effective the salon staff clean and disinfect foot spas, how often they are disinfected, and how the foot spas are maintained.

As a general and standard practice, a foot spa should be disinfected between each customer and nightly. Foot spas must be exposed to the disinfectants for the full time listed on their label, typically ten minutes depending on the type of disinfectant. Disinfectants used in the foot spa should indicate on the label that they are approved for hospital use. Therefore, if a foot spa aesthetician is not sure if a disinfectant is approved, it should not be used.

COMMON MICROBAL AGENTS IN SPAS AND SALONS

Some of the most common bacterial agents that arise a serious concern in beauty salons include *Staphylococcus aureus, Streptococcus,* and *Pseudomonas aeruginosa*. These bacteria enter the skin through cracks, wounds, burn injuries, insect bites, surgical incisions, or any types of skin openings. *Staphylococci* are gram-positive spherical bacteria that occur in clusters resembling grapes. *Staphylococcus aureus* and *Staphylococcus epidermidis* are significant in infecting humans. *S. aureus* settles mainly in the nasal passages.

However, it may be found regularly in the skin, the oral cavity, and the gastrointestinal tract. *S. epidermidis* is an inhabitant of the skin and comprises more than 90% of the resident aerobic skin flora, but frequently causes skin infections in compromised patients, including drug abusers, those on immunosuppressive therapy, AIDS patients, and patients with an attached medical device such as a catheter.

Pseudomonas aeruginosa is considered a normal, skin-natural flora. The bacteria normally live on human skin and in the mouth but are able to infect any tissue with which they come into contact. Due to the general innocuousness of the bacteria, infections occur primarily in compromised patients. Transmission often occurs through contamination of inorganic objects, resulting in ventilator-associated pneumonia and other medical device–related infections, such as those from catheters. The main route of entry is through compromised skin and causes dermatitis. Dermatitis occurs when skin comes into contact with infected water; for example, in swimming pools, hot tubs, or foot spas. The infection is very mild and is treated easily with topical antibiotics.

Skin infections caused by less common bacteria may occur in hospitals, nursing homes, and saunas or during ordinary activities such as gardening. These microbial agents lead to most common types of bacterial skin infections, including cellulitis, erysipelas, folliculitis, furuncles, carbuncles, impetigo, and secondarily infected dermatoses. Cellulitis infections can affect both the skin and the body in general. Folliculitis is a bacterial infection associated with hair follicles. Using contaminated whirlpools, swimming pools, and hot tubs may be common causes of folliculitis. Furuncles or boils is an infection that also develops via the hair follicle and results in folliculitis. They may appear as deep abscesses and secretions.

Figure 5.3. Dermatitis and boils

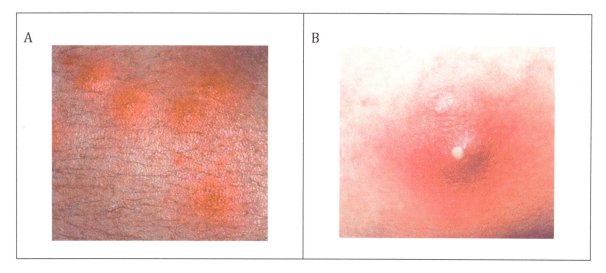

(A) Pseudomonas aeruginosa causes dermatitis when skin comes into contact with infected water; for example, in swimming pools, hot tubs, or foot spas. (B) Boils are firm red swellings about 5–10 mm across that are slightly raised above the skin surface. Boils are bacterial infections of hair follicles and the surrounding skin that form pustules around the follicle. Boils are sometimes called furuncles. When several furuncles merge to form a single deep sore with several "heads," or drainage points, the result is called a carbuncle.

TREATMENT FOR BACTERIAL INFECTIONS

Treatment for bacterial skin infections depends on the type and severity of the disease. Samples from the affected areas can be obtained and cultured in a laboratory in order to identify the bacteria. Blood tests and antibacterial sensitivity tests may also be performed to plan proper treatment strategies. Antibiotics may be applied to the skin in the form of creams, lotions, or liquids. Infections that have spread throughout the body are treated with orally taken/systemic antibiotics. People that are carriers of Staphylococcus aureus may use preventative antibiotics. Severe skin infections may require significant surgery and even skin grafts. In some cases, systemic infections can cause mental confusion or death. In addition to bacterial risks, people can develop viral or fungal infections in contaminated salons and spas.

FUNGAL INFECTION

Fungi usually grow in moist and dark areas of the body where two skin surfaces touch. Most common areas are between the toes, in the genital area, and under the breasts. Most of the fungi that infect the skin are present only in the stratum corneum, the topmost layer of the epidermis, and do not break through deeper. Overweight individuals are more prone to fungi infections due to excessive skin folds where skin meets. In addition, people with diabetes are more at risk for fungal infection. Surprisingly, fungal infections on one part of the body can produce rashes on other parts of the body that are not infected. For example, a fungal infection on the foot may cause an itchy, bumpy rash on the fingers. If a red, irritated, or scaly rash in one of the commonly affected areas is observed, fungal infection can be diagnosed and confirmed by scraping off a tiny area of the affected skin and having it examined in a medical laboratory through a microscope and/or a specific culture medium that allows the growth of fungus.

CANDIDIASIS

Candidiasis is and infection caused by the yeast *Candida* that may cause rashes, scaling, itching, and swelling. *Candida* yeast is normally found in the mouth, digestive tract, and vagina and usually causes no infection. Under certain conditions, however, *Candida* can overgrow on mucous membranes and moist areas of the skin. Typical areas affected are the lining of the mouth, the area between thighs and abdomen, the armpits, the skin under the breasts in women, and the skin folds of the stomach. Conditions that contribute to candidasis include heat, humid weather, tight synthetic underclothing, poor hygiene, inflammatory diseases (such as psoriasis) that occur in skinfolds, use of antibiotics or corticosteroids and other drugs that suppress the immune system, and in diabetic patients.

Antifungal creams that are applied topically or antifungal drugs given by mouth usually cure candidiasis. Prolonged treatment for other infections by taking antibiotics may develop into candidiasis since the normal floral bacteria that normally reside in the body are weakened and/or removed by the antibiotics, giving an opportunity for infective species to grow.

Corticosteroids or immunosuppressive therapy after organ transplantation can also lower the body's defenses against candidiasis. Inhaled corticosteroids, often used by people with asthma, sometimes produce candidiasis of the mouth. Pregnant women, cancer patients under chemotherapy, and obese individuals are more likely to be infected by *Candida*.

NAIL FUNGUS

Nail fungus, also known as onychomycosis or Tinea unguium is a fungal nail infection of the fingernails and toenails. It most often occurs in the toenails rather than the fingernails and affects more than thirty million people in the United States and about 10% of people worldwide. These fungal infections usually cause white or yellow discoloration and thickening and often softening of the nails. Infected nails may have an abnormal appearance but are not itchy or painful. Older people, diabetic patients, and people with poor foot circulation are predominantly prone to fungal infections.

Nail fungus or fungal fingernails is a difficult condition to treat and may often cause permanent damage to the fingernails and possibly nail loss. The nails are very effective barriers, which makes it very difficult for a superficial infection to invade deep in the nail. Unfortunately, once an infection has occurred, the same barrier protects the microorganism, making it difficult to treat. Infection associated with Tinea unguium can be spread through contact with an infected person or with surfaces (such as a foot spas and bathroom floors) where the fungus is present. In more severe infections, the nails thicken and appear deformed and discolored. Eventually, they may detach from the nail bed.

Figure 5.4. Nail fungus

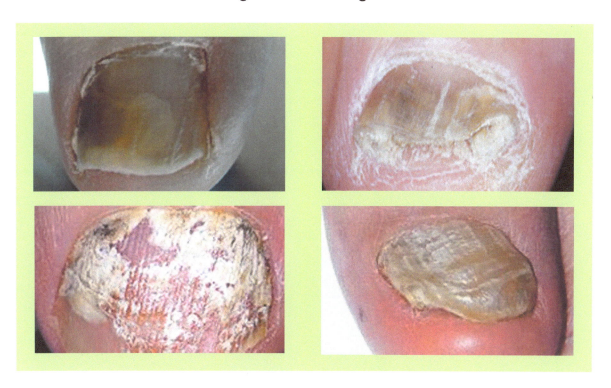

An infection of nail fungus occurs when fungi infect one or more of your nails. A nail fungus infection may begin as a white or yellow spot under the tip of your fingernail or toenail. As the nail fungus spreads deeper into nail, it may cause nail to discolour, thicken, and develop crumbling edges.

GREEN NAIL SYNDROME

Green nail syndrome is a nail infection caused by Pseudomonas aeruginosa, a motile, aerobic, gram-negative bacterium that grows optimally at thirty-seven degrees Celsius. The infection most often tends to occur in people whose hands are in prolonged contact with detergents or soapy water. The nails develop a mixture of greenish patterns. The area can be treated by soaking in a 1% acetic acid solution twice a day or by trimming back the nail and treating the area with an antibiotic solution.

It is very important to keep the nail dry. If the affected nail comes in the contact with water, it must be dried thoroughly. The bacterium survives in moist environments, therefore keeping the nail dry maybe an effective treatment against the bacteria. In addition, keeping the nail trimmed short can help greatly to cure the disease since it maintains the moisture lesser than long nails. Feet affected with green nail syndrome should be dried after bathing. In addition, absorbent socks should be worn and antifungal foot powder may be applied to the area. Old shoes may shelter a mass of fungal spores and should not be worn.

Figure 5.5. Green nail syndrome

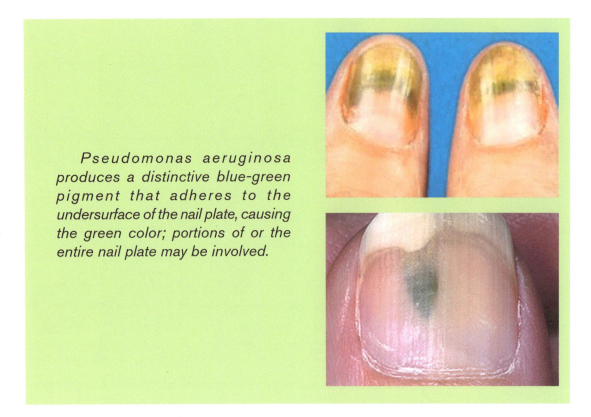

Pseudomonas aeruginosa produces a distinctive blue-green pigment that adheres to the undersurface of the nail plate, causing the green color; portions of or the entire nail plate may be involved.

TREATMENTS FOR NAIL FUNGUS

Underneath the nail is an optimal environment for the fungus to grow. Toenails are most affected by the fungus because they are especially prolonged in exposure to warm, moist, and dark conditions during daily activities. Socks and shoes must be cleaned and disinfected regularly. In severe infections, fungi often cause the area around the base of the nail to become red and irritated. Edges or base of the nail is the first location affected by the fungi. As the infection intensifies, the nail and nail bed show more visible changes.

Discolored yellow-green, dark yellow-brown, or white spots can be observed. There is often mild discomfort, itchiness, or even pain around the flesh surrounding the nails or cuticles. In progressed infection, the nails become brittle, jagged, and thickened and develop abnormal grooves, lines, and tiny punched-out holes. This condition may discourage the patient from social interactions. If left untreated, nail fungus can spread to other areas of the body and cause severe health threats.

Generally, a systemic boost in immune system can be substantially effective to prevent and/or eliminate fungal infections such as fingernail fungus. Nail fungus can infect people in public areas—such as locker rooms, swimming pools, or public showers where—bare feet are exposed. Because nail fungus is not highly contagious between people, factors other than exposure often must be considered. Many healthy individuals are exposed to fingernail fungus on a daily basis from other sources such as soil, water, or even in the air. A dermatologist can usually make the diagnosis based on the appearance of the nails. To confirm the diagnosis, a microbiology laboratory may perform microscopic examination of the nail debris sample and through medium culture to determine which fungus is causing the infection.

Nail fungus can be particularly unsafe to a person who suffers from diabetes, but it can become a complication for healthy individuals as well. In order to avoid a serious fungal infection or permanent nail damage, it is important that nail fungus be treated properly with an early diagnosis using an effective nail fungus medication. A prescribed nail fungus medication may be able to prevent the fungi from spreading beyond its initial occurrence. Some dermatologists may prescribe itraconazole or terbinafine as drug of choice.

Some physicians may recommend ciclopirox to people who cannot take oral drugs for other health reasons. Another most common nail fungus cure medications is known as leucatin. In order to determine if this, or any other, nail fungus medication is the right treatment method, the patients should ask their physician about potential side effects and whether or not the product can be an effective nail fungus cure based on their health condition.

FINGERNAIL FUNGUS TREATMENT BY LASER

Fingernail fungus can be treated with laser therapy in a short period of time. The procedure is safe, effective, and without discomfort. Clinical studies have shown about 88% effectivness rate, compared to prescription of topical cream treatments that only provide an 8% effectiveness rate after prolonged use. Since laser therapy is a drug-free procedure, it has no risk of side effects associated with prescribed drugs or oral treatments that require physician monitoring. Generally, the quick, effective laser procedure treats the nail without surgery and downtime.

INGROWN TOENAIL

An ingrown toenail is a condition in which the edges of the nail grow into the surrounding skin. An ingrown occurs when a deformed toenail grows improperly into the skin. Another condition that contributes to an ingrown toenail is when quick, abnormal growth of skin surrounds around or part of the nail. Wearing narrow and tight-fitting shoes and trimming the nail into a curve with short edges rather than straight across can cause or worsen ingrown toenails. Ingrown nails may appear first without symptoms, but in the longer period of time may become painful, especially when physical pressure is applied to the ingrown area. The area can become red, inflamed, and irritated. If left untreated, the area may develop infection. Once infected, the area becomes more painful, red, and swollen. Pus may accumulate under the skin next to the nail and lead to an infection of the cuticle called paronychia. For mildly ingrown toenails, sterile cotton may be placed under the nail following a gentle lift of the edge of the nail out from the surrounding skin until inflammation disappeared. If an ingrown nail requires further attention, the physician usually numbs the area with a local anesthetic and removes the ingrown section of nail.

Figure 5.6: Ingrown toenail

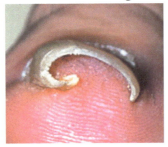
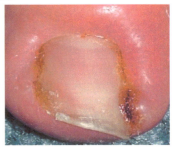

Ingrown toenail has grown into the skin instead of over it. This usually happens to the big toe, but it can also happen to other toes. An ingrown toenail can get infected. It may become painful, red, and swollen; and it may drain pus.

RISKS OF ACRYLIC/ARTIFICIAL NAILS

Aestheticians must ensure if there is any sensitivity to the materials in artificial nails before performing the procedure for their clients. It is highly recommended to have one nail done as a test and wait a few days to see if a reaction develops. If the natural nail or skin around it is infected or irritated, an artificial nail must not be applied until the infection heals. The ingredient list must be recorded in order to provide to physicians in case the client has an allergic reaction or other injuries. The artificial nails must be treated with care. Usually they are stronger than natural nail, but they still can break and separate upon applying too much force. However, the aesthetician has to make sure the client can perform ordinary tasks, such as using a pencil to dial or depress the numbers on the phone.

If an artificial nail separates, the fingertip should be dip into rubbing alcohol in order to clean the space between the natural and artificial nails before reattaching. This is necessary to prevent chances of infection. In order to reattach a separated artificial nail, household glues never should be used. Rather, only products intended for nails must be applied, and the directions must be followed with care. Artificial nails should not be worn for longer than three months at a time. It is for the ultimate benefit to remove them for one month to give nails a rest. Several clinical reports indicate that fungal infection can occur when an acrylic nail is left in place longer than three months since prolonged use of acrylic nails allows moisture to accumulate under the nail.

Bacterial and viral infections also can occur from using unsanitary nail implements, especially in a salon where the same implements are used on many people. Unclean implements are especially dangerous if the skin around the nail is broken. This can occur with manicuring in which the excess cuticle area is cut or pushed back too far. If the cuticle is cut or separated from the fingernail, infectious agents can get into the exposed area. It is highly recommended to leave cuticles intact. Common symptoms associated with finger infections are pain, redness, itching, and pus in or around the nail area. Yellow-green, green, and green-black nail discolorations are signs of a *Pseudomonas* bacterial infection. A blue-green discoloration signals a fungal infection.

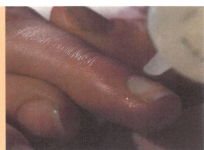

Figure 5.7

Removing acrylic nails can end up with sore, ridged, and generally unattractive nails.

chapter 6

Skin Rejuvenation Procedures

INTRODUCTION

BIOLOGY OF SKIN AGING

SKIN-FAT REDUCTION BY MESOTHERAPY

MESOTHERAPY PROCEDURE

TYPES OF MESOTHERAPY TECHNIQUE

DRUGS USED IN MESOTHERAPY

PHOSPHATIDYLCHOLINE

INTRODUCTION TO CHEMICAL PEELS

HOW CHEMICAL PEELS WORK

CHEMICAL PEEL PROCEDURES

GLYCOLIC PEEL

TRICHOLORACETIC ACID PEEL

BLUE PEEL

VITALIZE PEEL

LACTIC PEEL

SALICYLIC PEEL

RETIONIC ACID PEEL

PHENOL PEEL

MICRODERMABRASION

MECHANISM OF MICRODERMABRASION

- INTENSE PULSED LIGHT
- IPL PROCEDURE
- THERMAGE
- INTRACEUTICAL OXYGEN FACIAL
- MEDICAL SKIN NEEDLING
- MSN MECHANISM OF ACTION
- MSN TECHNIQUES

CHAPTER 6

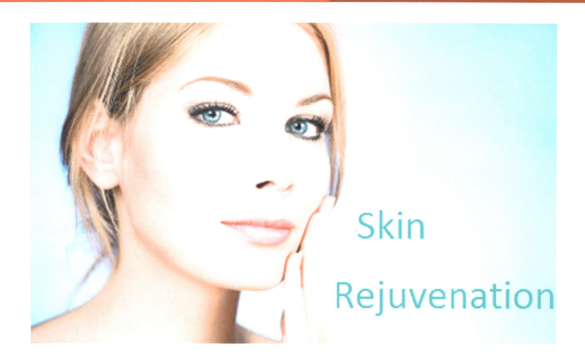

INTRODUCTION

Skin rejuvenation techniques are used to restore youthfulness and improve the appearance of aged or wrinkled skin. Skin biology and the biology of aging can help us to better understand the concepts of skin rejuvenation and to apply effective skin rejuvenation strategies. The skin is the body's most prevalent organ. It serves many important functions, including sensing stimuli, regulation of body temperature, and maintenance of water and electrolyte balance. In addition, the most critical functions of the skin are keeping vital chemicals and nutrients in while providing a barrier against pathogens, microorganisms, and foreign agents from entering into the body. It also provides a safeguard from the harmful effects of the sun's ultraviolet radiation.

A healthy skin plays a significant role in a happy lifestyle, beauty, and social interaction. Therefore, any factor that interferes with skin function or leads to changes in normal appearance can have devastating consequences ranging from physical illness to mental constraints. For example large brown aggregations and large collections of overconcentrated capillaries can give an aged-looking face and a red, plethoric, and rather spotty look that may affect one's social activities. An uneven, rough-textured complexion may give an impression of age and fatigue. On the other hand, many studies have shown that clear, translucent skin, regardless of color, is perceived as being young and attractive.

BIOLOGY OF SKIN AGING

As people age, several changes happen gradually to the dermis. The dermis makes up about 90% of the skin's thickness and contains key cellular and molecular elements implicated in the maintenance of healthy, young skin. Two important constituents of the dermis that significantly influence skin's healthy condition are collagen and elastin fibers.

Among different cell types that exist in the dermis, fibroblasts are major cells that regulate connective tissue homeostasis. This means that fibroblasts play a critical role in connective tissue repair and conservation, collage production and degradation, and overall extracellular matrix turnover and balance. Fibroblasts secrete different growth factors and proteoglycans that are crucial for keeping up the skin's healthy condition and repair process upon wounding. One of the most common signs of an aging dermis is the reduction in the number of cells, particularly fibroblasts. Reduced fibroblasts may affect skin regeneration and turnover. This often leads to reduced collagen and elastin fibers that result in the volume loss and rigid skin, respectively.

An aging skin undergoes a number of changes. One of the most important ones occurs in the connection between the dermis and the outermost layer of the skin, the epidermis, known as cell junctions. Cell junctions provide contact between neighboring cells and between a cell and its surrounding matrix and facilitate intracellular communications, transport of nutrients, and exchange of minerals. Cell junctions are especially abundant in the epidermis or epithelial tissues. As people age, these cell connections become flatter, leading to reduced nutrients and metabolic waste transportation.

Figure 6.1. Morphology of a fibroblast

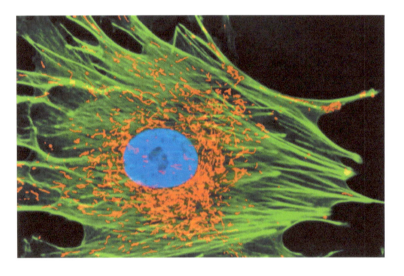

Dermal fibroblast cells synthesize the extracellular matrix and collagen, the structural framework for animal tissues that play a critical role in healing.

Figure 6.2. Structure of collagen fibers

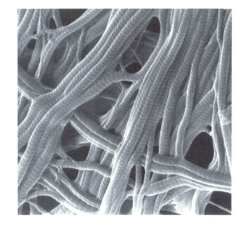

This is what type I collagen, a typical structural collagen, looks like. Observation of tendons under a powerful microscope reveals long, wavy bundles of fibers on the order of two to ten microns thick (a human hair is about fifty to a hundred microns). Like the fibers of a rope, these fibers are made up of smaller structures called fibrils. At this level, the precision of the collagen structure can be seen. Under an electron microscope, the fibrils appear long, smooth, and uniform. (In type I collagen, for example, all the fibrils are between fifty and seventy nanometers in thickness.)

The first consequence may be dry skin. In addition, the attachment between the layers becomes less firm. As the result, even a minor injury can cause the two layers to separate and skin blisters to occur more often. The blood vessels of the dermis also change, especially under the influence of excess sun radiation. The sun's UV rays may cause the thickening of blood vessels in the dermis. During the aging process, the blood vessels also become more dilated, leading to onset of the spider veins in older people. Excess exposure to the sunlight can also damage collagen and cause a severe reduction of skin elasticity. The outcomes manifest as wrinkles and folds and loss of softness or flexibility in the skin. In addition, prolonged exposure to the sun may lead to irregular pigmentation, brown and red spots, and the rough texture of the skin.

The aging of skin results in the thinning of the dermis and epidermis. The underlying fat can be lost as well. The decrease in volume and overall effectiveness of all three skin layers accelerates skin aging and results in a number of important medical and cosmetic effects. For example, loss of skin elasticity can make it drier due to decreased production of essential oils such as sebum. Another consequence of skin aging is reduction of the nerve endings and deterioration of sensation. The number of sweat glands and blood vessels decreases upon aging of the skin, leading to reduction of the skin's ability to respond to heat exposure. The number of melanocytes tends to decrease with aging, so the skin has less protection against ultraviolet radiation. All of these changes make the skin more susceptible to damage.

Figure 6.3. Skin aging

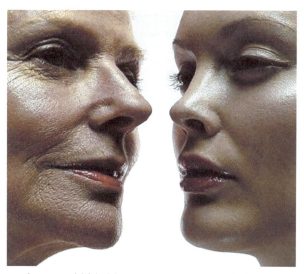

The skin changes as people age. Wrinkles, age spots, and dryness can be noticed upon aging. The skin also becomes thinner and loses fat, making it less plump and smooth. The healing process might take longer as well.

SKIN-FAT REDUCTION BY MESOTHERAPY

Traditional liposuction is a major surgical procedure that involves the removal of fat tissue through several small stab punches in the skin and a suctioning of the fat. In contrast, mesotherapy is a noninvasive procedure that is composed of a series of microinjections of specially selected drug(s), vitamins, and/or amino acids into the areas of the body where the unwanted fat deposit is located. Mesotherapy is a noninvasive alternative to liposuction that slowly dissolves the deposits with injections of fat-dissolving substances. Development of unattractive skin lumps and bumps is very common in all age groups. This uneven-looking skin feature is caused by excess deposit of adipose tissue (fat) under the skin. One effective method of skin fat reduction is mesotherapy. This method specifically targets localized fat and cellulite deposits.

Mesotherapy has been in use in France for more than fifty years, and its popularity is escalating in Canada and the United States. Over the last ten years, mesotherapy has been successfully practiced on thousands of people in South Africa and in South American countries. French physician Dr. Mihael Pistor is recognized as the pioneer of mesotherapy. During the course of a mesotherapy treatment, the body naturally eliminates the residue over the following three to four weeks. Four to fifteen treatment sessions may be required to accomplish the desired results.

Using injectable fat-dissolving substances to target cellulite and localized fat deposits has made mesotherapy advantageous for achieving body contouring without extensive surgery. Mesotherapy treatment consists of injections of natural soybean lecithin and enzymes in small quantities that break up the persistent fat deposits hard to remove by diet and exercise. In addition to vitamins, amino acids are injected into the fat underlying the skin. The procedure includes sequential injections into the intended areas of localized fat. Injection of lipolytic or fat-dissolving substances can also be used to reduce the size of unpleasant lipomas, smooth, round benign tumors of fatty tissue.

MESOTHERAPY PROCEDURE

Basically, the method of mesotherapy is performed without a general anesthetic. It has a very short recovery period, allowing a rapid return to work and normal activities. Mesotherapy is a safe procedure involving the delivery of fat-busting drugs directly into the unwanted fat deposits and, later on, the evacuation of the fat-waste through the body lymphatic system. In addition, compared to traditional surgical procedures such as liopsuction, mesotherapy is noninvasive and cost-effective. Results can be quickly seen in usually three to eight treatments.

Side effects such as temporary bruising, itching, and soreness are minimal and temporary. The results usually last for several years, providing the client maintains a healthy lifestyle and be physically active. Clients for mesotherapy need to manage their eating habit in order to prevent weight gain. After the treatment, there may be some swelling and discomfort that peaks at about 48 hours. Most people handle the discomfort with Tylenol.

Figure 6.4. Skin fat reduction by mesotherapy

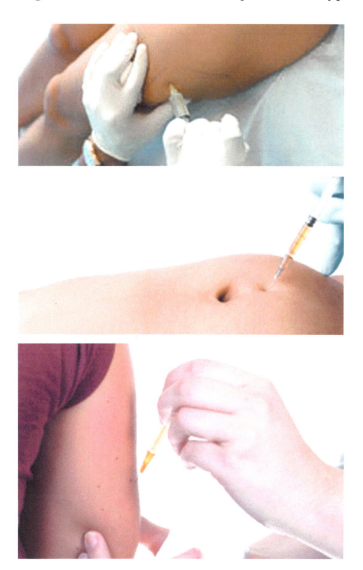

Lipodissolve or mesotherapy is an effective procedure for reducing fat or cellulite by injecting small amounts of soy lecithin and bile salt directly into areas that are too fat, such as legs, arms, abdomen, or thighs. The mixture injected destroys fatty cell walls, leading to the metabolization and excretion of the cell's content.

TYPES OF MESOTHERAPY TECHNIQUES

The procedure is most effective in patients who are not excessively overweight. The areas that react greatest to lipodissolve treatment are localized fat deposits that resist additional diminution after diet and exercise, such as in the backs of arms, thigh saddlebags, knees, love handles, certain areas in the abdomen, and the area on the back. There are many techniques of delivering these drugs, but two techniques are most popular:

Subcutaneous Microinjections

Subcutaneous microinjections are performed by a physician using a syringe with an extrathin needle attached. The therapist holds the fold of skin overlying the unwanted fat deposit and gently inserts the needle, which is a very short 6 mm in length. As the needle is very thin and sharp, there is very little discomfort during microinjections. The injections must be carefully done into the subcutaneous fat underlying the skin rather than injected mistakenly into the muscles.

Nappage Technique

In the Nappage technique, the drug composition is first distributed over the skin, followed by microinjections with a 4 mm mesotherapy needle. The *nappage* technique causes little discomfort that can readily be eliminated with a numbing cream applied earlier. MesoGlow is a form of mesotherapy that consists of a series of microinjections midway down into the skin. Not deep enough to draw blood, but enough to get nourishment to the skin. A series of droplets are put into and on top of the skin to start the process. MesoGlow can be used to cover the entire skin surface and in areas where injections are not possible, such as the upper and lower eyelids. MesoGlow compliments dermal fillers in these areas. The effects of MesoGlow rejuvenates the face, eyelids, and neck without the unnatural appearance and painful recovery of surgical facelifting. This is a popular treatment for fine lines around eyes and lips.

Figure 6.5. Needles used in mesotherapy

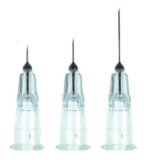

The ultrathin diameter of 27 g, 30 g, and 32 g mesotherapy needles make them excellent for the procedure. Sterile and disposable, the accurate sharpening of the needles minimizes the pain associated with treatment and ensures precision.

DRUGS USED IN MESOTHERAPY

The ingredients of the solution used for the mesotherapy injections depend on the purpose of the treatment. The most common elements are phosphaditylcholine (a fat-buster), vitamins, sodium deoxylate, and other microelements. Cellulite is treated with enzymes (hyalorunidase, collagenase) that target fibrous bands compressing fat tissue in the buttocks or thighs. Also, an anesthetic (lidocaine) is used to dilute the drug. These substances are FDA approved and injected directly into the fat to shrink the fat cells, essentially "dissolving" fat from unwanted areas. In general, there is a very low risk of allergic reaction from any of the drug components. Mesotherapy is generally very safe when performed in a medical office with an experienced physician.

PHOSPHATIDYLCHOLINE

Phosphaditylcholine (PC) is a natural compound derived from soy lecithin in a certified compounding pharmacy. Treatment of unwanted fat deposits is accomplished by the injection of minute quantities of PC (in concentrations of 50 mg/ml or 100 mg/ml) dissolved 1:1 with lidocaine (an anesthetic). PC is used in intensive care units for treatment of patients with fat emboli. The mechanism of action of PC involves lipolytic (fat-dissolving) activity by affecting the permeability of the adipocyte's (fat cell) membrane and subsequent fat mobilization. Compounding pharmacies add small quantities of sodium deoxylate into each vial of PC in order to increase the fat-busting effectiveness of PC. Sodium deoxylate is known to cause disintegration of the walls of fat cells.

Figure 6.6. Molecular structure of PC

Representation of the phosphatidylcholine molecule showing the choline head attached to the phosphate group, which is attached to the triglyceride shoulder. Two polyunsaturated fatty acid chains are also connected to the triglyceride shoulder. (Not shown to scale.)

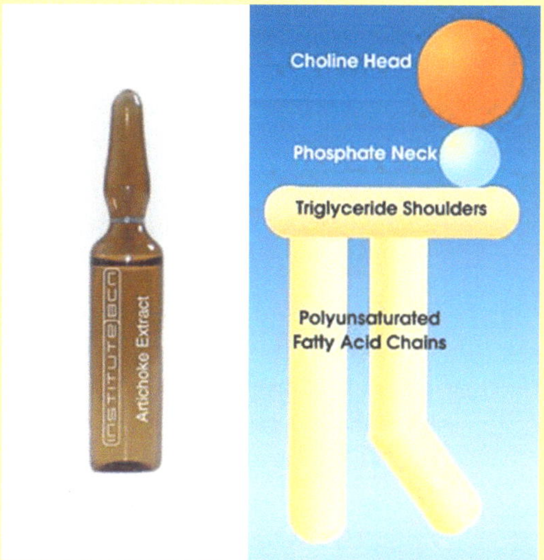

INTRODUCTION TO CHEMICAL PEELS

Chemical peels have been used for decades in medical cosmetology. They work by chemically removing the outermost layer of the skin and giving the skin a younger, healthier appearance. Chemical peels play a very important role in skin rejuvenation as they remove skin dullness, blotching, and age and sun spots and reduce fine lines and wrinkles. However, a chemical peel will not correct deep wrinkles or loose skin, but it is a rapid means of enhancing overall appearance. In general, they can be used as a standalone procedure or as a part of a combination treatment together with other procedures. Based on the goal of the treatment, a special chemical solution is applied for a very short period of time (a few minutes only) to exert a desired beneficial effect by removing the outermost layer of the skin or the deeper skin layers. Chemical peeling is a procedure performed in the office, after which the patient returns home.

There are three basic types of the chemical peels: superficial, medium and deep. The difference is associated with the depth to which they penetrate the skin. Chemical peels can be applied to face, neck, arms, hands, back, or legs. Over the years many different peeling substances have been used, and newer techniques and technologies now offer safe and effective ways to improve the texture of the skin.

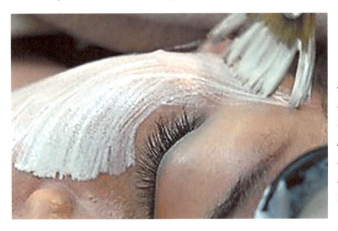

Figure 6.7. Chemical peel

A peel utilizes a chemical solution that is specifically designed to remove dead skin. Essentially, it "peels" away a layer of dead skin cells to reveal the smoother and less wrinkled skin below. Although going to a dermatologist is not required to receive this treatment, it should only be performed by a certified professional who has received proper training and has gained experience.

To perform the procedure, the skin must be cleansed to remove all oils, dirt, and soap traces. Then the peeling solution or solutions are carefully applied to the appropriate areas. For some, this may be a full face peel, which would cover the entire face. Others may need a partial peel, such as around the mouth to reduce fine vertical lines, for the forehead for diminishing the horizontal wrinkles, or on the cheeks for fine wrinkles and age spots. The treatment may be accompanied by some stinging or a mild burning sensation.

Depending upon the peel treatment, the skin may become somewhat red and a little swollen and flaky (similar to a sunburn) for a few days. About one in ten patients will have some brown patches, which peel off within seven to ten days. During the healing process, the cells that are shed are replaced by a fresh new skin surface. After healing, there may be some temporary mild pinkness that gradually fades, which can be covered up by makeup. People that have rosacea, pigmentation, and acne or those who want to rejuvenate their skin would all benefit from chemical peeling. However, the clients should undergo a careful assessment of skin type to determine which peel would be most suitable. Every peel also includes suggestions for proper home care and sun protection.

How Chemical Peels Work

The highlight of a chemical peel is its effectiveness at removing dead skin cells and yielding skin that is smoother in texture with more even pigmentation. Peels also cause new collagen to be produced, leading to a firmer skin and, eventually, a visible reduction in wrinkle depth, length, and number. Chemical peels provide a good solution for skin rejuvenation; reduction of fine lines and small wrinkles; reduction/removal of age spots, hyperpigmentation, sun damage, and melasma; and reduction of acne and acne scars.

However, a chemical peel is less likely to remove medium or deep acne scars or clear skin from acne if used as a standalone procedure. A combination therapy for skin rejuvenation may include microdermabrasion, photo-facials, or laser therapy together with chemical peel if medically indicated and if chemical peels are appropriate for a skin of a given client. An individual with very sensitive skin is not a good candidate for the chemical peels. Peels should be used in a series, sometimes in combination with prescription medications for the most benefit. Recovery time can range from a few hours to a few days, depending on the type of peel used, the strength of the solution, and the patient's needs.

Chemical Peel Procedures

The client who is undergoing chemical peels must be tested using a step-up approach. This requires that the strength of substances for peeling is gradually increased. A response of the skin to a peel applied previously will guide the practitioner in the pace of the treatments. After examination of the skin condition by a cosmetic physician, the skin care therapist must cleanse the skin, apply protective eye pads, and gently distribute a prescribed peel solution using a special brush. The peel will stay on the skin for a determined period of time (usually between three and five minutes) or until the end point of the treatment.

Then, the peel on the surface of the skin will be neutralized, and the chemical(s) will be removed from the skin by rinsing it thoroughly. At the end a gentle moisturizer and sunblock must be applied. The side effects may include a sensation of tingling to the skin during the application and a perception of skin tightness. Faces treated with chemical peels may be minimally pink for several hours after the treatment. Usually, four to eight sessions are needed for a significant effect, depending on the skin condition. Treatments are usually offered every ten to fourteen days or as needed. The candidate for chemical peeling must be instructed to stop any exfoliation procedures performed at home at least one week before the procedure, to wear a sunblock at all times, and to stop use any cream containing retinol or hydroquinone at least seven days before the first peel.

Glycolic Peel

The glycolic peel is a harmless, simple, and painless exfoliation process that removes damaged cells and a thin layer from the top of skin. Removal of damaged cells stimulates cell division that results in fresher and healthier young cells. A glycolic peel is comprised of an all-natural alpha hydroxyl acid derived from sugar cane. Alpha hydroxyl acids exist naturally in certain fruits and foods. The benefits of glycolic peels include improved skin texture, color, and tone; diminished fine lines; reduced acne; increased moisture content; and, to some extent, smoothed coloration and lightened hyperpigmentation.

The glycolic peel can be performed on the face, neck, chest, hands, and even the arms and legs. Patients usually note a burning sensation similar to sunburn after the procedure. As with any exfoliation or resurfacing, it is important to use sunscreens because the skin is more susceptible to injury by the sun. Mild glycolic acid–based peels take about twenty minutes. For optimal effect, it is recommended that glycolic peels are performed weekly for six weeks. Occasionally, patients with very sensitive skin may have mild temporary redness or irritation.

Tricholoracetic Acid Peel

A deeper, more active treatment, tricholoracetic acid (TCA) peels are ideal for patients with dramatic wrinkling, sun damage, and acne scarring. The peel consists of lactic acid, ascorbic acid (vitamin C), plumping phytohormones, and kojic and azelaic acids to produce dramatic results without the discomfort and downtime associated with traditional TCA peels. The concentration of the TCA is the only factor that determines the depth of the penetration and the possibility of side effect occurrence. The procedure includes the utilization of milder acids or other agents first, such as Jessner's solution or solid carbon dioxide. This allows use of TCA concentrations in the 30–35% range. These concentrations more deeply penetrate the skin since the other agent, prior to peeling, has removed the outer layers. TCA peels may be uncomfortable during the procedure.

Blue Peel

The Obagi Blue Peel was designed and formulated by dermatologist, Dr. Zein Elabdine Obagi. The Obagi Blue Peel has been suggested to be effective in lessening the blemishes, acne scars, wrinkles, uneven pigmentation, and sun damage. It may stimulate skin cell renewal and improve turnover and rebuilding of collagen. Using a low concentration of the TCA mixed with a special blue base to slow penetration, the Blue Peel allows monitoring of the appropriate depth to effectively remove the thin surface layers of and damaged skin from the face or other parts of the body. Some clients have reported freshly proliferated and healthier skin cells replacing dead skin cells, and a feeling of skin clarity and tightness is appreciated right after the procedure. Several peels may be necessary to give the desired result. In most cases, one to three Blue Peels can achieve improvements in many skin problems. The peels can be performed in six- to eight-week intervals until the desired goals are reached. Makeup should only be applied after the skin is completely healed.

Vitalize Peel

A Vitalize Peel is a combination of retinoic acids, alpha hydroxy acids, and rescorcinol. The Vitalize Peel has been suggested to clinically help pigmentation problems (such as age spots) and stimulate collagen production. It is also recommended for inflammatory acne. Compared to other peels, Vitalize Peel is much more aggressive. It may produce results faster, but it also leads to more redness and significantly more peeling between treatments. Vitalize Peel may be used if a quicker results is desired.

However, for patients who want a very gentle treatment with no downtimes and minimal discomfort and who do not wish to have heavy exfoliation and peeling for four days after the treatment, microdermabrasion or lactic treatment are a better choice. Patients who should avoid the Vitalize Peel include patients with a history of allergies, rashes, or other skin reactions, anyone with an allergy to salicylates, patients who have taken Accutane within the past year, patients who received chemotherapy or radiation therapy, pregnant or breastfeeding women, and patients under the age of twelve.

Lactic Peel

Lactic acid is derived from milk. It's frequently used, alone or in combination with other chemical peels, for light and medium skin peels. A Lactic Acid Peel is one of the most gentle and effective cosmetic chemical peels designed to exfoliate the skin while reducing the risk of irritation and redness. It promotes healthy skin and improves the appearance of fine lines and pigmentation. This treatment is ideal for rosacea and sensitive skin. Women who wish to continue their normal skin care routine during pregnancy can use lactic acid peels.

Salicylic Peel

Salicylic acid is an antibacterial, anti-inflammatory pore cleanser that works by dissolving surface oil. It diminishes blackheads and pimples by penetrating deep to clean out clogged pores. A salicylic peel is ideal for oily, acne-prone skin.

Retionic Acid Peel

This is derived from retinoids which is denatured vitamin A. This type of peel is much deeper than beta peels and is used to remove scars, as well as wrinkles and pigmentation changes. It is chemically similar to Retin-A and has a similar effect on fibroblasts, collagen-producing skin cells. Basically, retinoic acid peel is so effective that it stimulates active skin cells division. In addition, retinoic acid peel contributes to sealing moisture in the skin at the deepest level, stimulates collagen production, and has an antiseptic effect since retinoic acid inhibits the growth of various bacteria.

Phenol Peel

This is the strongest and deepest type of skin peel. The phenol is actually a carrier for another component in the peel, croton oil, which is the active ingredient. The effects of this peel are extremely long lasting (up to twenty years) and a single treatment can usually be sufficient to obtain the desired results. This is the deepest peel. It is administered under carefully monitored conditions due to the possibility of effects on the heart, as well as the fact that anaesthesia is often required due to the pain. Phenol peels are not used as much as they have been in the past due to developments of other peels that are less unbearable and obtain the same results.

MICRODERMABRASION

Microdermabrasion is a skin-freshening technique that helps to polish the skin, especially in the facial area. It can alleviate fine lines; pigmentation; acne; and dull, dry skin. It is believed that microdermabrasion stimulates the production of skin cells and collagen. It is also used to remove the rough skin of keratosis pilares found on the upper arms and shoulders. Microdermabrasion is a noninvasive treatment in which natural mineral crystals are gently forced on the surface of the skin for placid epidermal abrasion. Its detaching action on the damaged and unhealthy epidermis promotes the skin's repair mechanism to produce epidermal growth resulting in skin quality and softness. The exfoliation of the skin using microdermabrasion can improve the appearance of aging skin, fine lines, scarring, sun damage, and wrinkles. The procedure works on all skin types without risk.

Mechanism of Microdermabrasion

Microdermabrasion involves gentle blowing of fine sand or crystal particles against the skin. The application wand then sucks up the particles to remove them from the surface of skin. The sand particles used in microdermabrasion cause a very mild abrasion to the skin, causing detachment of damaged or dead layers of epidermis and a clearing of the pores of debris. During a microdermabrasion treatment, nylon and silk coats are moved across the skin with applied vacuum suction, resulting in a very gentle and controlled exfoliation of the skin.

Multiple treatments fade pigment away and surface irregularities, such as fine wrinkles and acne scars, begin to soften. When epidermal cells turn over, they provide a younger and healthier skin. Some microdermabrasion systems use a stream of fine mineral crystals that move over the skin polishing it smoothly and safely. It is relatively a fast procedure with little or no discomfort. For example, treatment of the whole face takes about thirty minutes. The treated area may be slightly pink for one to two days. For most skin disorders, a minimum of six treatments can provide highly satisfactory results. Results can be seen in both the texture and the appearance of the skin after one or two sessions.

Figure 6.8 Mechanism of microdermabrasion

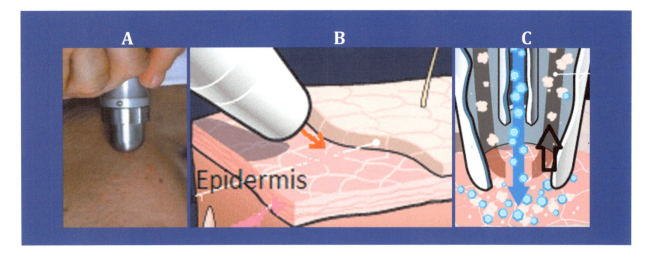

(A) Microdermabrasion is a skin-freshening technique that helps to polish the skin, especially in the facial area. (B) Microdermabrasion involves a gentle blowing of fine sand or crystal particles against the skin (red arrow). (C) The application wand then sucks up the particles to remove them from the surface of skin (black arrow).

Figure 6.9

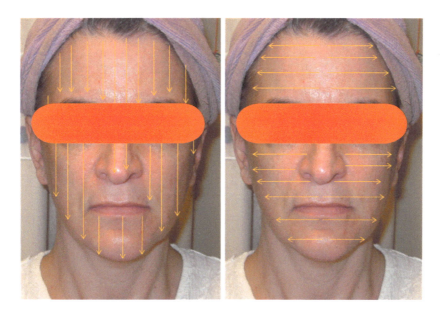

Direction of microdermabrasion wand in two runs of the procedure

INTENSE PULSED LIGHT

Intense pulsed light (IPL) was first designed to strip the paint off airplanes. It has, however, been refined and adapted to a great extent and currently represents one of the greatest advances in the treatment of aging skin. Pulsed light can deliver hundreds or thousands of colours of light at a time. Pulsed light machines use "cut off" filters to selectively deliver the desired wavelengths. These wavelengths can be customized to reach the specific hair, blood vessels, or skin component being treated and can be modified with each pulse. Pulsed light begins with all wavelengths of light from 500 to 1200 nanometers (nm)—including green, yellow, red, and infrared light. Various lower range cut off filters (ranging from 515–755) block light shorter than the wavelength of the cut off filter. Since longer wavelengths penetrate deeper into the target, it is used to treat deeper targets and to avoid and protect superficial parts of the skin.

An experienced practitioner of a pulsed light device can adapt settings to select the wavelengths, number of pulses, duration of pulses, delay between pulses, and the power delivered to best match the relative depth, size, and absorption characteristics of the intended target. Thus, the settings that may cause damage to the areas that need to be conserved can be avoided. These enhanced capabilities can thereby be used to target the larger and deeper hair follicles, and spare the superficial melanin in darker skin types by utilizing longer wavelengths, and larger beams for deeper penetration.

IPL Procedure

The procedure starts with pretreating skin with a cooling gel. Then, a handheld device emits small intense bursts of light on the skin. Light is absorbed to varying degrees depending on the surface color. Therefore, darker areas are targeted, absorb the light differentially, heat up, and are thereby broken down. The procedure is continued until all the abnormal skin has received the small pulses of light. The penetration depth and heat intensity is controlled to minimize complications. The light energy that is applied to the skin is very effective in reducing both red and brown pigments, and some of the longer wave lengths also stimulate new collagen formation so that the face becomes more coherent and luminous rather than dull and spotted.

IPL is considered an effective technology for skin rejuvenation, correction of sun damage, improvement of skin tone, and reduction of pore size and unwanted superficial vein treatment. It destroys unsightly blood vessels by sending very short pulses of light into the skin, destroying the vein using heat. The vessels shrink over the following weeks and are reabsorbed by the body.

Figure 6.10. Intense pulsed light

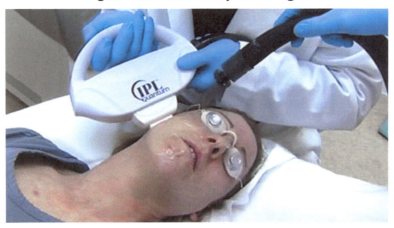

Intense pulsed light works by delivering precise amounts of light energy through the skin's surface using a specialized handpiece. The light energy is absorbed by the target tissue (redness, brown spots, or both), resulting in disruption of the unwanted skin color. Over time, redness and brown spots will begin to fade, leaving skin to look more vibrant and rejuvenated. In addition, the light energy stimulates production of natural collagen, which helps improve large pore size, fine lines, and wrinkles.

LEVULAN PHOTODYNAMIC THERAPY (LPDT)

Levulan, a prescribed drug also known as ALA, is a colorless photosensitizing liquid with 20% aminolevulenic acid. The treatment is based on special properties of Levulan that upon application over the skin surface, is slowly absorbed by the outermost layer of the skin, and then activated by special blue light with wavelengths of 419–420 nm known as BLU-U. LPDT treatment removes sun-damaged areas on the skin called actinic keratoses. Fine lines and blemished pigmentation can also be corrected by this treatment. LPDT is effective in minimizing pores, reducing oil glands, and treating acne and rosacea. It also improves the appearance of some acne scars.

The dermatologist or cosmetic physician can determine the number of treatments in a personal consultation and assessment session. The side effects may be redness and peeling skin for up to seven days. There may also be temporary swelling of the lips and around the eyes. Some dark spots may be intensified in color. As Levulan is a photosensitizing agent, it is crucial to avoid sun exposures for at least twenty-four hours following the treatment. Using sunscreen may dramatically reduce the risk of side effects.

Levulan combined with IPL treatments considerably enhances the appearance of skin. LPDT can also be performed in conjunction with microdermabrasion. Used for acne treatment, Levulan is especially effective in the destruction of bacterial agents responsible for acne onset. Microdermabrasion prior to LPDT may help to unclog pores and remove blackheads and whiteheads, as well as exfoliate the surface of the skin. The photodynamic acne treatment program typically consists of three PDT treatments that are performed once a month.

THERMAGE

Skin Tightening by Thermage

The technology of Thermage was invented in the United States and successfully introduced to more than seventy countries. The Thermage procedure originally was developed for providing a nonsurgical facelifts and neck lifts, but it has been utilized to tighten the skin on the body and eyelids. It is also currently used for nonsurgical brow lifts and the nonsurgical tightening of facial wrinkles on the forehead, around the eye, and the middle and lower face. Thermage reduces the signs of aging skin by actually tightening the underlying tissue. It is a safe, noninvasive, and clinically proven way to tighten and shape the skin without incisions.

The improvements in tone, contour, and texture occur naturally through the stimulation of body's own collagen. Thermage treatment utilizes radiofrequency energy to heat up the collagen in the lower layers while the top layers of skin are protected with a cooling spray. This deep volumetric heating causes the skin to tighten and new collagen to grow, which results in enhancing facial contours, tightening the skin, and producing a more youthful appearance. The treatment can take up to three hours. Results appear gradually in two weeks to six months. Results can last for years, depending on the skin condition and aging process. Minor side effects and complications that can occur include mild redness or swelling and, extremely rarely, transient blistering of the skin.

Figure 6.11. Principle of Thermage technology

The Thermage technology uses radiofrequency to lift and tighten sagging skin. This radiofrequency gently heats the deep surface of the skin, causing it to contract and tighten.

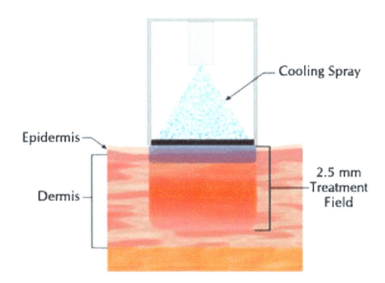

Adopted from http://www.technologyofbeauty.com/thermage.cfm

INTRACEUTICAL OXYGEN FACIAL

Intraceutical oxygen facials involve a combination of oxygen technology and restorative relaxation. These exceptional skin care treatments concurrently infuse moisture, vitamins, and antioxidants into the skin using cool, calming, topical, hyperbaric oxygen. Using a natural aminopeptide complex clinically proven to smooth the dermis and significantly diminish the appearance of fine lines and wrinkles, the intraceutical oxygen facial treatment can be used for sun or environmentally stressed skin. It is reported that intraceutical treatments also speed up healing time and reduce sensitivity after IPL treatments, photodynamic therapy, and pixel treatments. The oxygen infusion system uses therapeutic-grade oxygen under pressure to infuse a skin specific cocktail of hydrators, essential vitamins, botanicals, antioxidants, and amino peptides to the deeper layers of the skin.

MEDICAL SKIN NEEDLING

Clinical studies have suggested medical skin needling (MSN) to be as effective as laser resurfacing, dermabrasion, and chemical peels. It is suggested that MSN acts comparably to IPL or Fraxel treatments in stimulating collagen and elastin production in order to thicken the skin. The most common conditions that can be treated with MSN are wrinkles and fine lines, loss of skin elasticity, acne, surgical scarring, stretch marks, hyperpigmentation, and hair loss prevention and/or restoration.

The resulting effect may improve wrinkles and stretch marks and smooth acne scars. MSN, also known as collagen induction therapy (CIT), works by stimulating the body's own collagen production to reduce the appearance of fine lines, wrinkles, stretch marks, lax skin, and scarring such as that caused by acne or chicken pox. It has also been successfully applied to the indication of hair restoration in cases of alopecia.

MSN Mechanism of Action

Medical skin needling involves introducing a series of fine, sharp needles into the skin following the administration of a topical local anesthetic to reduce discomfort. The needles are attached to a sterile single-use roller that is moved over the surface of the skin to create many microscopic channels or columns, approximately 0.07–0.25 mm wide, at various depths of penetration (2–3mm). In the case of medical rollers, this is within the papillary dermal layer of the skin where collagen and elastin fibers are located.

This controlled damage to the dermis encourages the body to produce new collagen and elastin, which stimulates skin cells (fibroblasts) to accurately repair themselves, thus the skin becomes more voluminous and fleshier and thus appears more youthful. Although primarily used on the face, this procedure can be carried out anywhere on the body, such as on stretch marks, on the thighs and abdomen, and generally on all skin types. Cosmetic rollers for home use reach a much shallower level in the epidermis (about 0.3mm), where they aid absorption of topical ingredients. These minute punctures close over almost immediately as the skin heals.

MSN Techniques

Preparation for the medical skin needling includes the application of vitamin A and C topical lotions for a minimum of two weeks prior to the performance of the procedure. A similar skin care regime will also be recommended for up to six months posttreatment to support the healthy production of the new collagen and the rejuvenation of the skin. Treatment sessions with medical-grade rollers take between ten minutes and an hour, depending on the size of the area being treated. Pain should be minimal due to the application of the topical anesthetic.

Usually, the skin appears pink or red in appearance for about two hours following the treatment. Some minor superficial bleeding may occur depending on the treatment level, the length of needle used, and the number of times it is rolled across the treatment area. Side effects usually include minor shedding or dryness of the skin, some small white spots, and hyperpigmentation. Most patients are able to return to work the day following the treatment.

Recovery time depends on the treatment level and the length of the needles. It can take between three and ten weeks before visible signs of skin rejuvenation are observed, and the process will continue over the following months. A single treatment can produce noticeable results; however, a package of two to five treatments performed every two months is often recommended to achieve optimum results. Medical skin needling treatment is suitable for most skin types. However, it is not recommended for patients with open wounds, cuts, or abrasions to the skin or have received radiation treatment within the last year.

People with herpes simplex (cold sores), or any other infection or chronic skin condition in the area to be treated, and those who have areas of the skin that lack sensation are not good candidates for MSN. Pregnant or breast-feeding women should not be treated with MSN. People with a history of keloid or hypertrophic scars or poor wound healing should not choose medical skin needling for skin rejuvenation.

Figure 6.12. Medical skin needling

A

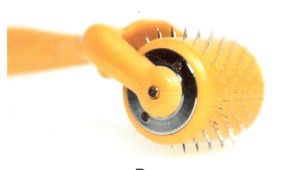

B

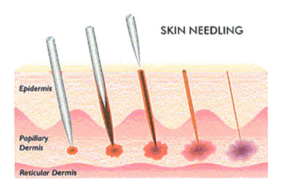

C

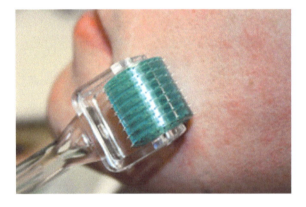

Medical skin microneedling is a method (A) by which multiple puncture wounds are made in the skin penetrating in to the papillary and reticular dermis (B) in order to stimulate new skin cells, angiogenesis, and collagen. The indications for micromedical skin-needling are acne scars, traumatic scars, wrinkles, fine lines, aged and sun-damaged skin, pigmentation, dilated pores, sebum overproduction, and stretch marks (C).

chapter 7

Laser Cosmetics

DEFINITION

LASERS' MECHANISMS OF ACTION

TYPES OF LASER COSMETICS

CO2 LASERS

RUBY LASERS

ND-YAG 1064-NM AND 532-NM LASERS

ERBIUM LASERS

ERBIUM VS. CO2 LASERS

PULSED-LIGHT LASERS

ALEXANDRITE AND Q-SWITCHED LASERS

DIODE LASERS

PULSED DYE LASERS

HOLMIUM LASERS

LASER-COOLING MECHANISMS

LASER HAIR REDUCTION

FITZPATRICK SCALE

BEST CANDIDATES FOR LASER HAIR REMOVAL

ELECTROLYSIS VS. LASER HAIR REMOVAL

TYPES OF HAIR REMOVAL LASERS

LASER HAIR REMOVAL: RISKS AND SIDE EFFECTS

- LASER HAIR REMOVAL: BEFORE AND AFTER
- LASER TATTOO REMOVAL
- MECHANISMS OF LASER TATTOO REMOVAL
- LASER AND SKIN REJUVENATION
- LASER SKIN RESURFACING
- LASER LIPOLYSIS (LIPO LASER)
- LASER HAZARDS CLASSIFICATION
- LASER SAFETY

CHAPTER 7

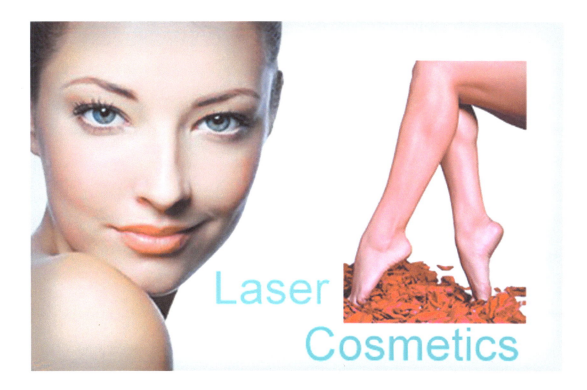

DEFINITION

The word *laser* stands for light amplification by stimulated emission of radiation. Laser therapy can be used to treat a variety of normal and pathological conditions. Several cosmetic laser systems are available in the market for the treatment of various skin conditions, such as hair removal, facial wrinkles, acne and acne scars, surgical scars, moles, melasma, stretch marks, and sun damage. Compared to chemical peels, cosmetic laser therapy has been found to be better tolerated by patients and cause little discomfort. The side effects are transient and include discomfort sensations like a prickly heat during treatment.

In addition, a facial bronzing and puffiness associated with laser treatment may occur that lasts for a few days. Different types of lasers emit specific colors of light and are used to treat various cosmetic and surgical problems. The laser light is generated by a monochromatic light emission from a low-intensity laser diode or an array of high-intensity superluminous diodes. The monochromatic, coherent, and polarized characteristics of the light beam permit penetration of deep tissues. The particles of light energy that are absorbed by a variety of micromolecules within the cell initiates a number of physiological responses.

LASERS' MECHANISMS OF ACTION

Lasers used in medical aesthetics operate at different wavelengths on the electromagnetic spectrum. Laser light with longer wavelengths penetrate the skin deeper while at the same time allowing effective treatment for people of all skin colors, even those with darker or black skin. In contrast, lasers with a shorter wavelength can only treat fair-skinned people, but may be more effective in treating fine hairs. The effect of laser therapy also depends on pulse duration, which is the length of time that a defined amount of energy is delivered to the target tissue. Longer pulse durations allow the skin to heat up slower and are safer for darker skin tones. Alternatively, shorter pulse durations can be more effective for treating fine and light-colored hair.

Lasers vary to as great an extent as the pulse durations available, which dictate the amount of energy given to a defined location. The amount of energy delivered to a given area is referred to as fluence. However, while higher fluences will achieve better hair removal results, it may raise the risk of thermal damage. Operator experience is extremely important in delivering a laser with optimal fluence in order to achieve effective results without side effects.

All laser devices have also a standardized spot size. Spot size determines the area to be treated. Lasers vary widely on the spot sizes available, which are chosen for a particular treatment. For example, a spot size of at least 3–5 mm is required for effective hair removal. Spot size also determine the depth of penetration. The larger the spot size, the greater the depth of penetration. Thus, an optimal spot size provides effective hair removal with minimal thermal damage. Smaller spot sizes are still useful because the operator can use higher fluences. The larger the spot size of the laser beam, the more fluence must be used to achieve the same result. Lasers have limits as to the amount of energy that can be used with the larger spot sizes. Another advantage of the larger spot size is the ability to treat larger areas of the body very quickly. Based on the scientific and clinical principles, there is not one laser that can treat everyone. Also, the ability to manipulate the settings on each laser needs an extremely fine balance.

TYPES OF LASER COSMETICS

There are many kinds of lasers available, which each have a specific range of effectiveness depending on their wavelengths and penetration. The lasers are usually named for the amplification materials used. For example, the carbon dioxide laser is called a CO_2 laser while the YAG laser contains a solid material made up of yttrium, aluminum, and garnet. Many medical studies have shown that long-pulse, long-wavelength lasers provide the broadest range of treatment flexibility for all colors of skin, for the removal of unwanted hair, and for the treatment of varicose veins.

Other lasers—including ruby, alexandrite, and diode lasers—cannot penetrate as deeply with sufficient energy to be effective because the lasers' energy is absorbed at the surface of the skin. Some systems have a wavelength of 1064 nm, providing the maximum output energy 80 J—the highest available in an Nd:YAG laser, which is absorbed more slowly by both melanin and hemoglobin, ensuring that its energy can penetrate deeply to reach both hair follicles and varicose veins even in the darkest skin types. Below is the summary of medical lasers used in dermatology and cosmetology:

1. *Gas Lasers:* carbon dioxide, argon, copper vapor, etc. These are the first lasers that emit a constant beam of light for longer durations of exposure.
2. *Solid-State Lasers:* ruby, Nd:YAG, Er:YAG, KTP, alexandrite, etc. These emit interrupted emissions of constant laser energy.
3. *Liquid Lasers:* dye lasers. Pulsed dye lasers emit high-energy laser lights with very short pulse durations and longer intervals between each pulse.
4. *Diode Lasers:* diode lasers have several wavelengths and are suitable for soft tissue procedures.

CO_2 LASER

The carbon dioxide laser (CO2 laser) is one of the most common lasers used in surgery and is good for precise cutting and vaporizing tissue, that needed in the treatment of superficial lesions or the removal small volumes of tissue. The CO2 laser is a specialized laser that is filled with carbon dioxide gas and uses an infrared emission for cutting tissue through heat absorption. It is one of the earliest gas lasers, that was developed in 1964. CO2 lasers are the highest-power continuous wave lasers that are currently available with high efficiency.

The CO2 laser produces a beam of infrared light with the principal wavelength bands centering around 9.4 and 10.6 micrometers. Low cost and high power levels have made CO2 lasers popular. They are frequently used in industrial applications. CO2 lasers are very useful in surgical procedures and cosmetic laser surgery, such as skin resurfacing and dermabrasion, that involves thermally inducing the skin to promote collagen formation in the areas of treatment. The CO2 laser is also used by ophthalmic plastic surgeons to remove fine wrinkles from around the eyes. This laser precisely removes the outermost layer of skin and the underlying dermis, allowing the regrowth of wrinkle-free new skin.

Figure 7.1. laser's depth of penetration

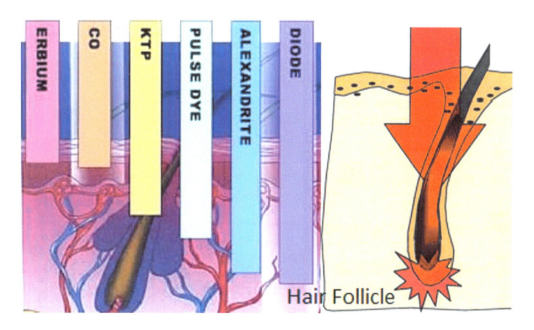

There are several different types of medical lasers used in dermatology and cosmetology. Their effectiveness depends on their wavelength and depth of penetration.

RUBY LASER

The ruby laser is a solid-state laser that uses a synthetic ruby crystal as its gain medium. Ruby lasers produce pulses of visible light at a wavelength of 694.3 nanometers, which is a deep red color. Ruby is an aluminum oxide crystal in which some of the aluminum atoms have been replaced with chromium atoms. Chromium gives ruby its characteristic red color and is responsible for the lasing behavior of the crystal. This is the oldest type of laser used for hair removal purposes. Ruby laser is suitable for those with fair or white skin and works best for light and fine hair types, whereas it is not a laser of choice for candidates with tanned or darker skin. Ruby lasers also cover a relatively smaller area than other lasers and, hence, has become popular for laser hair removal.

ND-YAG 1064-NM AND 532-NM LASERS

Nd:YAG stands for neodymium-doped yttrium aluminium garnet. $Nd:Y_3Al_5O_{12}$ is a crystal that used as a lasing medium for solid-state lasers. This laser may also be called a neodymium-YAG or ND-YAG laser. The dopant, triply ionized neodymium typically replaces yttrium in the crystal structure of the yttrium aluminium garnet (YAG) since they are of similar size. These lasers are used extensively in the field of cosmetic medicine for laser hair removal and the treatment of minor vascular defects, such as spider veins on the face and legs. Recently used for dissecting cellulitis, a rare skin disease usually occurring on the scalp. In laser eye surgery, the YAG laser is commonly used to vaporize a portion of the capsule, allowing light to pass through to the retina. The procedure is effective in eliminating the cloudy condition.

ERBIUM LASER

Erbium lasers produce energy in the midinfrared invisible light spectrum and is then to fifteen times better absorbed by water in the skin than the energy from CO_2 lasers. High degree of absorption enables the laser to precisely and instantly vaporize the target spots in the skin and tissue so that surrounding skin is barely affected. For this reason, the erbium laser has gain popularity due to its painless nature and minimal to no side effects, while the degree of precision and control is significantly enhanced. The erbium laser is generally used in skin resurfacing and is able to remove finer wrinkles with less damage to the skin.

ERBIUM VS. CO_2 LASER

The erbium laser is considered to be more precise and accurate than the CO2 laser. The depth of erbium laser penetration is about five microns, compared with the twenty microns typical of the CO2 laser. The erbium laser has also been shown to cause less uneven skin pigmentation in darker-skinned individuals since it creates a thinner laser area and less heat. The erbium laser has minimal heat diffusion and reduced tissue thermal damage; therefore, it has lower healing time than that with the CO2 laser. The erbium laser is frequently used in clinical procedure to emulsify the eye's natural lens during cataract surgery. Most cataract surgeons currently use a piece of equipment called a phacoemulsifier to break up and remove the cloudy lens. The erbium laser was chosen for the new technique because of its high absorption rate in water, a primary component of the eye's natural crystalline lens.

PULSED LIGHT LASERS

Intense pulsed light (IPL) is a technology meant to generate light of high intensity during a very short period of time. IPL was a treatment that first designed to strip the paint off airplanes. It involves a constructed xenon flash lamp and focusing optics together with capacitors whose rapid discharge provides the high energy required. The focused, broad-spectrum light is applied to the surface of the skin by way of either a handheld wand or an articulated arm.

The IPL technology represents one of the greatest advances in the treatment of aging skin because the light energy that is applied to the skin is very effective in reducing both red and brown pigments and some of the longer wavelengths also stimulate new collagen formation so that the face becomes more coherent and luminous rather than dull and spotted. This light travels through the skin until it strikes the target within the tissue, such as hair shafts or the bulb of the hair. The pulses of light produced by IPL equipment are very short in duration, so discomfort and damage to nontarget tissues is minor. IPL technology is also employed in the treatment of aging skin, sun-damage induced dyspigmentation, vascular changes, acne rosacea, and vascular and pigmented birth marks.

ALEXANDRITE AND Q-SWITCHED LASERS

Quality-switched systems in which ultrashort bursts (10 to 100 ns) of stored high energy are produced include the 694-nm ruby laser, the 755-nm alexandrite laser, and the 1064-nm Nd:YAG laser. The longer wavelength of these lasers makes them most appropriate for the treatment of dermal pigmented lesions. Q-switching, which is often called giant pulse formation, occurs when a laser creates high-powered pulses of light. The result is a laser beam that emits pulses of light that are extremely concentrated and powerful.

DIODE LASER

A laser diode is a laser where the active medium is a semiconductor similar to that found in a light-emitting diode. The way Diode Laser Hair Removal works is that when the laser beams are thrown on to the specific area, the energy of the beams heats up the pigment called melanin in the skin. Devices, which are most commonly employed in this method, include the SLP 100, F1 Diode, Light Sheer, MeDioStar, LaserLite, Epistar and Apex 800. Because this laser uses a longer wavelength of light in its working it is more effective on people with darker skin.

PULSED DYE LASERS

A dye laser uses an organic dye as the lasing medium, usually as a liquid solution. Compared to gases and most solid-state lasting media, a dye can usually be used for a much wider range of wavelengths. The wide range of frequencies makes them particularly suitable for pulsed lasers. In addition, the dye can be replaced by another type in order to generate different wavelengths with the same laser, although this usually requires replacing other optical components in the laser as well.

Dye lasers are very versatile. In addition to their recognized wavelength agility, these lasers can offer very large pulsed energies or very high average powers. Flashlamp-pumped dye lasers have been shown to yield hundreds of joules per pulse, and copper laser–pumped dye lasers are known to yield average powers in the kilowatt regime. The pulsed dye laser delivers energy at a wavelength and duration that has been optimized for the selective treatment of vascular lesions. Pulsed dye lasers have been used as an alternative to surgical excision or carbon dioxide lasers.

HOLMIUM LASER

Also known as the infrared holmium YAG laser, the holmium laser is used in a refractive surgery procedure. The holmium laser is perhaps the most versatile surgical laser available to today's laser surgeon.

Because of the unique ability of the holmium laser to vaporize, ablate, and coagulate soft tissues at relatively low depths of thermal penetration; its excellent hemostasis; and its delivery systems that allow access to even the tightest of spaces, the laser has encouraged many practitioners to apply the laser in their practice. Holmium laser energy, at 2100 nm (2.1 microns), is rapidly absorbed by the water in tissue and has an ultimate depth of penetration of 0.4 mm or less. Holmium laser energy can ablate hard materials such as calcified urinary tract calculi while also being able to treat the delicate structures encountered in spinal, gynecological, and ENT surgery.

Figure 7.2 shows those wavelengths between approximately 700 and 1000 nanometers (nm) are selectively absorbed by melanin; the competing chromophores (oxyhemoglobin and water) absorb less energy at these wavelengths. Therefore, any light source that operates between 700 and 1000 nm is appropriate for targeting melanin in the hair shaft.

Figure 7.2

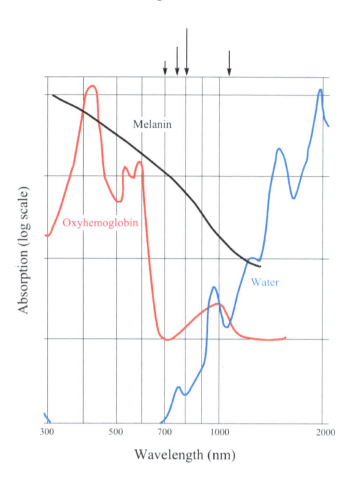

Adapted from J. L. Boulnois's "Photophysical Processes in Recent Medical Laser Developments: A Review," published in Lasers in Medical Science, vol. 1, 1986

LASER-COOLING MECHANISMS

Since laser light is converted to thermal energy when it reaches the target, cooling mechanisms are needed to prevent thermal damage or burns. Therefore, most laser devices in medical aesthetics are equipped with a cooling mechanism necessary to prevent damage to the surrounding cells where no treatment is needed. Generally, through diffusion of heat during skin laser therapy, the temperature exposed to melanin pigment may be increased in the hair follicle beyond its capacity and/or dispersed into the surrounding structures. Cooling mechanisms protect the surface of the skin and decrease the risk of blistering and unwanted pigment alteration. In addition, they cause less pain and swelling and more effective results. The generation of extreme heat on darkly pigmented skin can also be controlled effectively with cooling mechanisms.

There are several basic types of cooling mechanisms used with lasers. Cryogen-, air-, and contact-cooling systems are examples of advanced technology with minimal adverse effects. Cryogen spray is the most common method of cooling in lasers. Cryogen is a refrigerant at -30 to -50°C that is sprayed onto the skin before and/or after laser irradiation. It distributes consistent and effective cooling on the skin treated by the laser. However, in addition to being costly, excess cryogen spray may cause skin freezing and blisters. Air-cooling mechanisms can be an effective alternative with minimal side effects.

The application of cooling gels is the least effective cooling mechanism due to uneven distribution of the gel during the procedure and potentially insufficient cooling. It also provides short-term, superficial effectiveness and may be unpleasant to some users. Contact-cooling can be very accurate and effective. This method uses a cold gliding handpiece over a gel. The most important consideration for a client in medical spa settings is to choose an experienced cosmetic physician or a licensed technician who is knowledgeable in different laser and cooling methods. The laser operators must also be very skillful with the technique used, especially if contact cooling is the preferred cooling method.

LASER HAIR REDUCTION

Hair removal lasers have been successfully used in the cosmetic industry for several years, providing satisfactory results for the clients. Lasers target terminal hairs with the pigment melanin, thereby the intense pulse of the laser beam is absorbed primarily by the pigment in the hair follicle. Each light pulse lasts for only several thousandths of a second, so the energy from the beam is almost completely absorbed by the hair bulb without significant spreading to the surrounding tissue. Terminal hairs are thick, long, and usually pigmented with melanin. Hair on the scalp, underarms, genitals, eyebrows, chest, back, legs, and arms are examples of terminal hairs. Short and nonpigmented hairs that can be found in most other areas of the body and face are called vellus hairs.

Age, ethnicity, weight, metabolism, medication, and hormones all play a role in the location, resilience, and thickness of hair. Lasers destroy hairs by targeting the bulge and papilla region. The light energy from the laser is converted to thermal energy in the hair follicle. This process is referred to selective photothermolysis. It is selective because it targets only the hair and not the skin. Photo means "light," and thermolysis means "destroying with heat." The bulge area of the hair follicle is involved in the hair cycling and regeneration, while the papilla is the vascular structure of hair follicle and is associated with nutrition and O2 supplementation. Without normal follicles, hair cannot survive and falls down. In addition, lasers are most effective when targeting the hair follicle in its active phase of its growth cycle (called anagen). Destroyed hairs are then either dissolved within the skin or rejected by the body within the next several days. The hair shafts themselves will fall out within three to four weeks after the treatment.

A successful laser hair-removal program in achieved by repeated treatment since only a portion of all hairs in the body are in the anagen phase at any given time. This varies in individuals and in different areas of the body, usually from 20 to 85% of total hair. Some follicles are destroyed, while others are partially traumatized, reduced to fine hairs or subjected to extended quiescence. Generally, about 30% of the hairs will not regrow after a single treatment. It is difficult to predict how many treatments each individual will require to achieve the best long-term benefits. Therefore, multiple treatments are needed to provide the best results.

The FDA has approved laser treatment for permanent hair reduction, but not permanent hair removal, which is endorsed by many cosmetic clinics. It is possible that with a sufficient number of treatments, true "permanent hair removal" can eventually be achieved. Taken together, after all the laser sessions have been completed, it takes approximately six months before one can make a final judgment regarding the success of the treatment.

FITZPATRICK SCALE

The Fitzpatrick Classification Scale was developed in 1975 by Harvard Medical School dermatologist, Thomas Fitzpatrick, MD, PhD. This scale classifies a person's complexion and their tolerance of sunlight. It is widely used by many practitioners to hair type for laser treatment and to determine how someone will respond or react to facial treatments.

Figure 7.3 demonstrates the Fitzpatrick skin type that is governed by genetic factors and does not change throughout their lifetime despite changes in facultative pigmentation (tanning). Physicians administering laser or photo (light) therapy must first assess the patient's skin type to determine the appropriate dose—that is, the amount of exposure—which will provide beneficial effect whilst minimizing damage incurred. Similarly, researchers examining skin conditions need to cater their experimental design and treatments to individual variations in skin type.

Figure 7.3

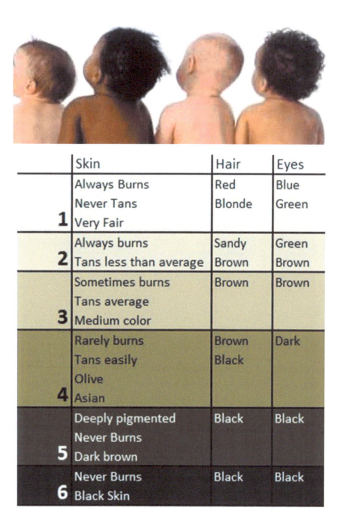

	Skin	Hair	Eyes
1	Always Burns Never Tans Very Fair	Red Blonde	Blue Green
2	Always burns Tans less than average	Sandy Brown	Green Brown
3	Sometimes burns Tans average Medium color	Brown	Brown
4	Rarely burns Tans easily Olive Asian	Brown Black	Dark
5	Deeply pigmented Never Burns Dark brown	Black	Black
6	Never Burns Black Skin	Black	Black

BEST CANDIDATES FOR LASER HAIR REDUCTION

People with coarse dark hair and light skin color respond the best to laser hair treatments. In clients with darker skin color who have more melanin in their skin, the skin tends to compete with the hair to absorb the light energy, resulting in potential damage to the skin. It is strongly recommended to avoid tanning before any laser treatment program. People with grey hair are the most difficult to treat as less energy is absorbed by the hair roots. All parts of the body can be treated with the exception of the area immediately surrounding the eyes. In women, the most common areas are underarms, bikini line, chin, upper lip, arms, and legs. In men, the most common areas are the back, shoulders, and the beard area.

Lasers can be used individually or in combinations for different skin and hair types to produce the best results. Treatments can be performed without anesthesia. There is some pain because the individual hair follicle is surrounded by nerve endings. While clients may be able to tolerate the procedure without the use of an anesthetic, others may find the application of an anesthetic cream helpful. A generous layer of anesthetic cream is applied for sixty minutes before the procedure and can provide adequate relief from discomfort during the procedure.

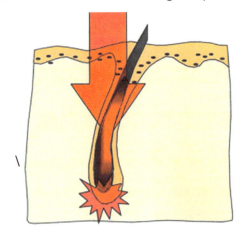

Figure 7.4

Absorption of the light occurs in the melanin in the hair shaft. The hair follicle reaches a temperature sufficient to cause irreversible thermal damage whilst the epidermis has remained below the damage threshold.

ELECTROLYSIS VS. LASER HAIR REMOVAL

Electrolysis treats one hair at a time by inserting a fine probe into what is hopefully the base of the hair and destroys the hair root using small electric shocks. Unlike electrolysis, the laser uses a wide beam, which treats many hairs at once. However, electrolysis is useful in removing hairs from small areas, such as the area around the eyes and in the nose. Laser hair removal is not only faster than electrolysis but can treat hairs that are untreatable by electrolysis. The laser offers a permanent reduction in the amount of hair and also, often, a reduction in thickness and color of the hairs that may grow back. Long-term studies have indicated that all the hairs that respond to the laser are permanently destroyed, thus the laser is considered the treatment of choice for those who desire to reduce their unwanted hair for a long period of time.

In certain circumstances, there may be persistent hairs that may take several treatments before they are destroyed. A realistic expectation is an 80–90% hair reduction. Often any remaining hairs are finer and lighter than they were previously. At least two weeks prior to laser hair reduction program, waxing, plucking, threading, electrolysis, and bleaching should be avoided. Makeup can absorb laser energy and interferes with its effect; therefore, it is important not to wear makeup when a facial laser procedure is performed.

TYPES OF HAIR REMOVAL LASERS

Alexandrite, diode, and Nd:YAG are the three prevalent types of hair removal lasers made by a range of manufacturers. In order to ascertain the most appropriate device to use, first an assessment of the client's skin type according to the Fitzpatrick scale is necessary. This system is based on a person's response to sun exposure in terms of the degree of burning and tanning the individual experiences. Below is the summary of the Fitzpatrick classification:

Type 1: Highly sensitive, always burns, never tans. Example: red hair with freckles or albinos.
Type 2: Very sun sensitive, burns easily, tans minimally. Example: fair-skinned, fair-haired Caucasians.
Type 3: Sun-sensitive skin, sometimes burns, slowly tans to light brown. Example: darker Caucasians, European mix.
Type 4: Minimally sun sensitive, burns minimally, always tans to moderate brown. Example: Mediterranean, European, Asian, Hispanic, American Indian.
Type 5: Sun-insensitive skin, rarely burns, tans well. Example: Hispanics, Afro-American, Middle Eastern.
Type 6: Sun insensitive, never burns, deeply pigmented. Example: Afro-American, African, Middle Eastern.

Alexandrite lasers are best for skin types 1–3 while diode lasers are best for skin types 1–4. Nd:YAG lasers are best for skin types 4 and darker. This is the only type of laser that should be used on skin types 5 and darker. Using any other types of lasers on this type of skin can result in burns if they are used at settings that disable the hair permanently. Intense Pulse Light systems (IPLs) are also used for hair removal. Some of the more popular brands of devices currently on the market are

(1) alexandrite: GentleLASE, Apogee;
(2) diode: LightSheer, F1 Diode, MeDioStar, Palomar SLP 1000, Comet (w/RF technology);
(3) Nd:YAG: CoolGlide, GentleYAG, Lyra-i, Sciton;
(4) alexandrite/ND:Yag Combination Devices: GentleMAX, Apogee Elite, Apogee MPX; and
(5) IPL: Palomar Starlux and EsteLux, Harmony, EpiLight, Aculight, Vasculigh, Aurora (w/RF technology).

LASER HAIR REMOVAL: RISKS AND SIDE EFFECTS

Some people may experience potential temporary side effects such as itching and redness for up to three days, swelling around mouth or follicle for up to three days, tingling, or a feeling of numbness. However, crusting and scab formation, bruising, purpura or purple coloring of the skin, temporary pigment change (including hypopigmentation or hyperpigmentation) are indicative of inappropriate laser type and/or settings.

LASER HAIR REMOVAL: BEFORE AND AFTER

The hair needs to be in place in order to be targeted by a laser as laser devices targets the pigment in the hair. Therefore, candidates for laser hair removal should not wax, epilate, or remove hair with the root using any other hair removal method for at least six weeks prior to their first session and throughout their course of treatments. The area to be treated should be shaved 1–2 days prior to treatments. This is critical for a successful procedure, as the laser energy should target the hair follicle instead of being worn out on the hair above the skin's surface.

Treating unshaved skin can result in burning of the skin by singed hairs. After the treatment, applying ice packs and cooled pure aloe vera gel is recommended. It is expected that all hair to shed within three weeks following the treatment. During the shedding phase hair may look like it's growing, but it is actually coming out to shed. Exfoliating and/or scrubbing gently in the shower can help speed up the shedding process. After three weeks, some patients may see small black dots remain in the hair follicles on some areas. These are commonly referred to as "pepperspots," which eventually shed on their own. Exfoliating may help speed up the process. Once new hair grows in, patients should come in for their next session. For most people and on most body areas, this happens about 8–12 weeks after the previous treatment.

LASER TATTOO REMOVAL

While tattooing has been popular among a number of people, studies have shown that at least 50% of people with tattoos would like to remove them due to different reasons. Many individuals that appreciate tattoos and have many of them on their skin may become tired of the old ones and would consider removing them and perhaps acquiring new tattoos.

Fortunately, laser tattoo removal is the safest, quickest treatment available with minimal side effects. Laser tattoo removal is the least of other more traditional methods of tattoo removal with a very low risk of scarring. Other treatment options for tattoo removal involve painful surgical excision and dermabrasion. However, they are rarely used today due to the longer recovery, the high possibility of developing scars, and the costs involved. Tattoo removal is a selective thermolysis procedure that delivers laser energy to the carbon particles or dyes that are found in skin tattoos, allowing selective destruction of the foreign pigment while minimizing damage to the surrounding skin. Lasers may be used on professional, amateur, cosmetic, medicinal, and traumatic tattoos. The different colors present in the tattoos may respond differently to laser tattoo removal.

Figure 7.5. How tattooing works

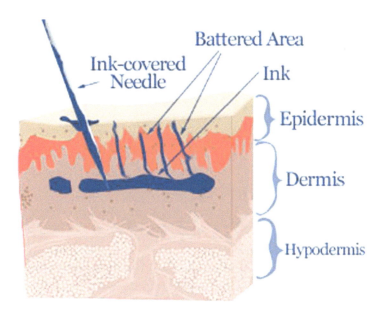

When you look at a person's tattoo, you're seeing the ink through the epidermis or the outer layer of skin. The ink is actually in the dermis, which is the second layer of the skin. The cells of the dermis are far more stable than the cells of the epidermis, so the tattoo's ink will stay in place, with minor fading and dispersion, for a person's entire life.

MECHANISMS OF LASER TATTOO REMOVAL

Tattoo removal by laser involves targeting the pigments by laser beam during multiple sessions. The pigment colors of the tattoo will break with a high-intensity laser beam. The light fragments the ink particles and the body absorbs these particles naturally. Tattoos generally require three to eight treatments for complete removal. However, the number of treatments varies with the individual and depends on many factors, including size, color, and depth of the tattoo; its location; and its age. Several weeks is needed between sessions of laser treatment. After each session, the tattoo becomes lighter. The color fades over a few weeks.

Many patients tolerate the removal procedure without freezing the sensation. A topical anesthetic can be applied to alleviate any discomfort if required. Determining which tattoo ink is used, how deep it is, or how much of it was used helps to clear it as quickly as possible. Black tattoo pigment absorbs all laser wavelengths, making it the easiest to treat. Dark blue and dark green ink can be removed the best as well. However, light red, light greens, and yellows are the hardest to remove. The newer tattooing devices place the ink deeper, and therefore, the tattoo is harder to remove whereas the older tattoos are easier to remove.

Side effects of laser tattoo removal include redness, mild swelling or tenderness, crusting, a sunburn sensation, or itching right after laser treatment. Side effects may also manifest as hyperpigmentation, infection, or pinpoint bleeding. Treated skin is sensitive and should be protected from sun exposure. An antibiotic ointment can be applied following the treatment and the area can be covered with a protective dressing.

Figure 7.6. Laser tattoo removal

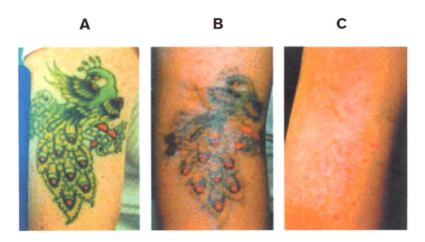

Laser therapy can be used to fade and remove tattoos (A–C). Most colors can be removed. Yellow, green, and white inks are difficult to remove. During the treatment, a laser is scanned over the tattoo and rapid pulses of light enter the pigment, breaking up the color, which is then absorbed by the skin and excreted by normal bodily functions.

LASERS AND SKIN REJUVENATION

There are a large number of cosmetic skin-resurfacing procedures that can be performed by laser therapy for nonsurgical skin rejuvenation and the improvement of aged and sun-damaged skin. Cosmetic lasers have now proven to give a smooth, glowing complexion after treatment of conditions such as photoaged, pigmented, wrinkled, or lax skin by stimulating collagen production. Laser therapy is also effective in treating acne and the resultant scarring. This treatment is noninvasive, has no side effects, and is suitable for all body areas including the face neck, chest, and back acnes. The high-intensity band light source penetrates both the skin surface and ducts to destroy acne bacteria and unclog congested skin. Laser therapy is also very efficient for removing unattractive, superficial visible veins and spider-like blood vessels.

LASER SKIN RESURFACING

Laser resurfacing is a major rejuvenation procedure. It is an efficient and inexpensive way to refurbish the younger appearance and freshness of the aged skin. The most preferred benefits of laser skin resurfacing are the considerable diminution of wrinkles, the obliteration of skin blemishes, and the elimination of sun damage, age spots, and sun spots. Certain types of scarring and most medium-depth wrinkles can be removed with laser rejuvenation.

Laser eyelid surgery has also become more popular since it treats tired, baggy eyes; drooping eyelids; wrinkles; crow's feet; puffiness; and dark circles with less bleeding and swelling and less risk of scarring compared to traditional surgical procedures. Skin resurfacing works by removing the outmost layers of skin (epithelium) until the wrinkles or scars are eliminated. Most clients can feel a fresh and rejuvenized skin three to five days after the treatment after reepithelilalization process is completed when new epithelium grows again. Laser resurfacing requires skill and the ability to follow up the patient in order to avoid any complications. Two types of lasers used for skin rejuvenation are called ablative and nonablative lasers.

The ablative lasers are those that utilize carbon dioxide or erbium (also known as microlaser peels) are very powerful lasers that remove the outermost layer of the skin up to 0.1 mm or 100 μm. Erbium:YAG Laser in combination with the CO2 Laser delivers a short burst of extremely high-energy laser light. The treatment requires a rapid one to two weeks healing process, after which skin rejuvenation is satisfactorily achieved by a smoother tighter appearance. After healing, there is a pink to red color that will fade over a few weeks to months.

One of the advantages of the erbium laser is that the preciseness that allows the depth of penetration is highly controlled. The erbium laser is highly absorbed by tissue water, and less heat is transmitted to the surrounding tissue. People with wide range of skin characteristics including darker skin can be treated with this type of laser. This procedure requires determination of the skin type and highly experienced practitioners to set the device appropriately for skin resurfacing.

LASER LIPOLYSIS (LIPO LASER)

The Lipo Laser has been approved by FDA and Health Canada as a noninvasive, painless laser treatment for spot fat reduction and aesthetic body contouring. The Lipo Laser's treatment is considered one of the most effective methods to reduce the appearance of cellulite and improve body contour. The Lipo Laser targets fat tissue layers in any areas of the body, including waistline, arms, legs, thighs, buttocks, and back. Lipo Laser is a nonsurgical adipose treatment, which reduces accumulated fat in fat cells called adipocytes (such as cellulite). It brings the broken down fat to the muscular layer where blood capillary flow is well distributed. Broken fat is then absorbed in the blood stream and naturally excreted.

Combining a healthy diet and regular exercise provide best results after a Lipo Laser procedure. At the cellular level, during treatments, the fat cells become permeable by laser. When the laser radiates on the fat cells or adipocytes, the contents of the cells move out of the cell membrane, become liquefied, and can be easily removed from the blood. The breakdown of fat cells is known as lipolysis, a process that converts fat to free fatty acids, water, and glycerol—which in turn are further processed through the body's natural metabolic functions.

Figure 7.7. Representative images of fat laser lipolysis

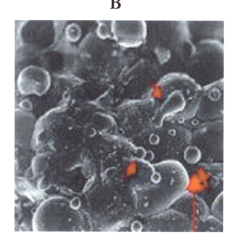

A   B

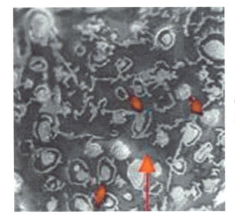

(A) Lipolysis by laser targets healthy adipose cells. (B) Fat droplets seeping across adipose cell membrane during laser treatment. (C) Complete collapse of adipose cell (emulsification).

LASER HAZARDS CLASSIFICATION

> The safety of lasers is classified into four groups:
>
> Class I: No known biological hazard.
> Class II: Chronic viewing hazard only.
> Class III: Direct viewing hazard.
> Class IV: Direct and reflected hazard.

1. Helium-neon lasers are class III. Dye, Nd:YAG, alexandrite, and diode lasers are class IV lasers and are dangerous to view due to scattered radiation. The use of goggles is mandatory.
2. All windows in a laser treatment room should be protected from beam transmission and covered with opaque material. There should be no mirrors in the treatment room.
3. All doors to a laser treatment room are to be closed and have a laser-specific danger sign along with a pair of laser-safe eyewear prominently displayed.
4. Eyes of patients and health care workers should be protected from laser beams. Laser-safe eye protection with appropriate wavelength and optical density should be worn by all health care workers and all patients and labeled to protect against improper use.
5. CO_2, erbium, or diode exposure may result in corneal absorption while pulsed dye, Nd:YAG, and alexandrite exposure may result in retinal absorption.
6. Patient eyewear choices include opaque tanning bed eyewear, laser eyewear with proper wavelength protection and optical density, or in the event neither are available, alternative eye protection may include moist sponges or a wet towel.
7. Flammable or combustible materials such as anesthetics, prep solutions, drying agents, ointments, plastics, resins, and hair should not be exposed to the laser beam.

8. How to deal with a plume: a plume is any smoke by-product from the laser's thermal destruction of tissue (may include skin, blood, or viral particles) and may be hazardous to one's respiratory tract. Plume can contain toxic gases and vapors such as benzene, hydrogen cyanide, formaldehyde, bio-aerosols, and dead and live cellular materials (including blood fragments and viruses). A laser-safe protective mask (0.1 m) should be used to decrease inhalation of particulate matter.
9. A laser should always be in standby mode unless an operator is ready to use it.

LASER SAFETY

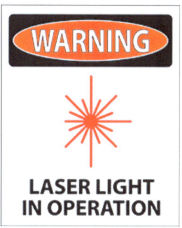

Figure 7.8.
Laser warning sign

Lasers used for hair removal are safe to use when specific guidelines are followed. Type IV laser devices are extremely powerful and all precautions must be taken to prevent unintentional exposure to the skin or eyes or direct or indirect reflected laser light. The wavelength for lasers used in hair removal can pass through glass or windows and can be reflected off metallic surfaces. Even though some of the lasers may use invisible light, it can cause permanent damage. Both the operator and the patient must wear protective eyewear appropriate for each piece of machinery. Even with protective eyewear, it is advisable never to look directly into the handpiece, laser beam, or scattered light from reflective surfaces.

It is now standard care to avoid laser treatments around the eye, including eyebrows. Treatment room doors should remain closed during treatments to prevent accidental exposure. Treatment room windows and portholes should be covered with a material of sufficient optical density to prevent laser light from escaping. Reflective objects, such as mirrors, should be removed from the treatment room. Warning signs should be posted in prominent locations. The exterior housing of a laser should never be removed, except by an authorized service representative.

Extremely high voltages can cause fatal shock. It is possible for the high voltage components to retain charge even after the laser has been turned off. Oxygen and flammable substances should not be used. This includes alcohol, acetone and flammable anesthetics. Patients must always remember to wear the appropriate eyewear provided to them and never take it off during treatment.

chapter 8

Facial Muscles Anatomy and Physiology

FACIAL MUSCLES AND MEDICAL AESTHETICS

PHYSIOLOGY OF MUSCLE CONTRACTION

NEUROMUSCULAR JUNCTIONS

FACIAL MUSCLE ANATOMY

CHAPTER 8

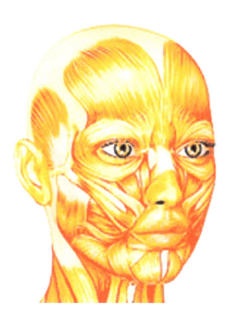

Facial Muscles: Anatomy and Physiology

FACIAL MUSCLES AND MEDICAL AESTHETICS

Facial muscles contracting at different times and to different degrees generate facial expressions. Excess facial muscle contractions contribute to many undesired facial wrinkles and folds that may be cosmetically unattractive and misinterpreted as being angry, concerned, sad, or tired. Selective weakening of the particular facial muscle or group of muscles that are responsible for the unwanted, wrinkled areas improves the overall facial appearance. However, in medical cosmetic procedures targeting the muscles responsible for the facial expressions and movements requires good understanding and knowledge of facial muscle anatomy as well as muscle physiology.

Figure 8.1. Facial expression

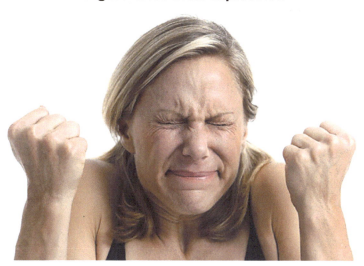

A facial expression results from one or more motions or positions of the muscles of the face. These movements convey the emotional state of the individual to observers.

PHYSIOLOGY OF MUSCLE CONTRACTION

Muscles produce tension and force by the act of contraction. Both the contraction and relaxation of different muscles are necessary to make each posture of the body. Muscles are an assembly of fibers enclosed together into large packs. Each fiber is made up of thread-like myofibrils. The basic units of contraction are called sarcomeres, which span the length of myofibrils. Proteins called Z-bands link sarcomeres to each other. There are two groups of filaments that contract within the sarcomeres known as myosin and actin. Small heads that extend from the myosin are placed only a billionth of a meter away from the actin, making it possible for myosin and actin to interchange locations along the sarcomeres. A small gap between the myosin and the Z-bands at the end of the sarcomere called I bands facilitate the contraction once the Z-bands are pulled closer to the myosin.

Actin is attached to both ends of the Z-band, with a little gap in the middle called the H zone. These gaps make it possible for, upon a muscle contraction, drawing actin filaments close to each other without contact. During the process of contraction, called the sliding-filament model, muscle contraction is initiated when motor neurons send signals to the muscle cells. The signals stimulate the release of calcium from the associated cell compartment (called the sarcoplasmic reticulum).

Increased levels of calcium expose sites on the actin to which myosin heads can bind. These heads slope in the direction of the center to draw the actin leading to the contraction of the sarcomere and, subsequently, the entire muscle. The myosin heads free their grasp on the actin when they bind with adenosine triphosphate (ATP). ATP is a transporter for chemical energy, which is produced in the metabolic course of action. Thus, after relaxation, the sarcomere is free to contract once more.

NEUROMUSCULAR JUNCTIONS

Neurons have elongated protrusions called axons, which terminate in dendrites, a bundle of fibers that can transmit chemicals to the next neuron. Neurons are specially designed cells that communicate using chemicals called neurotransmitters. The axons of motor nerves meet the muscle in the neuromuscular junction, where they convey signals from the nervous system leading to the muscle contraction and relaxation. Depending on the type of cell, specific neurotransmitters stimulate a response.

The neurotransmitter specific for the muscle function is called acetylcholine. It is the only neurotransmitter used in the motor division of the somatic nervous system as well as the principal neurotransmitter in all autonomic ganglia. At a neuromuscular junction, the surface of the muscle fiber forms small crumpled folds for the end of axon to fit in, where acetylcholine receptors are present. The neuron forms synaptic vesicles that are filled with acetylcholine. The synaptic vesicles look like small bulbs that release the neurotransmitter when the muscle needs to contract (Figure 8.3). One neuron can control many muscle cells, but each muscle cell only responds to one neuron.

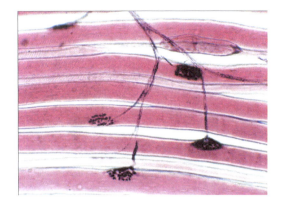

Figure 8.2. Neuromuscular junctions

The axons of motor nerves meet the muscle in neuromuscular junction where conveying signals from the nervous system leading to the muscle contraction and relaxation.

Figure 8.3. Schematic illustration of a neuromuscular junction

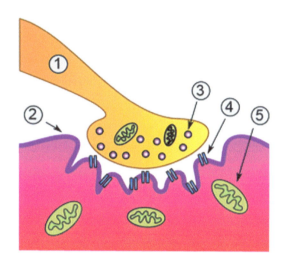

1. **Presynaptic terminal**
2. **Sarcolemma**
3. **Synaptic vesicle**
4. **Nicotinic acetylcholine receptor**
5. **Mitochondrion**

FACIAL MUSCLE ANATOMY

The facial muscles are a group of striated muscles innervated by the facial nerves that control facial expression. The facial muscles resemble elastic sheets that are stretched in layers over the cranium, facial bones, cartilage, fat, and other tissues of the head. The facial muscles may act individually and in combination to make the facial expressions. Facial muscles include, but are not limited to, the following: occipitofrontalis, procerus, nasalis, depressor septi, orbicularis oculi, orbicularis oris, corrugator supercilii, auricular, depressor anguli oris, depressor labii inferioris, risorius, zygomatic major, zygomatic minor, levator labii superioris, levator labii superioris alaeque nasi, levator anguli oris, buccinators, and mentalis.

Below, the location and function of each facial muscle is described:

Occipitofrontalis: the occipitofrontalis or epicranius is a muscle that covers parts of the skull. It consists of two parts: the occipital belly near the occipital bone and the frontal belly near the frontal bone. Supported by the occipital belly, the frontal belly draws the scalp back, which helps to lift the eyebrows and wrinkles the forehead.

Procerus: the procerus is a small pyramid-shaped muscle deep with the superior orbital nerve, artery, and vein. It helps to pull that part of the skin between the eyebrows downward, which assists in flaring the nostrils. It can also contribute to an expression of anger and produce transverse wrinkles.

Nasalis (compressor naris): the nasalis is a sphincter-like muscle of the nose that constricts the nasal cartilage. The depressor septi lies between the mucous membrane and muscular structure of the lip. The depressor septi is a direct antagonist of the other muscles of the nose, drawing the ala of the nose downward and thereby constricting the aperture of the nares.

Orbicularis oculi: the orbicularis oculi is the only muscle in the face capable of closing the eyelids. Loss of function for any reason results in an inability to close the eye. This condition may require frequent use of eye drops and, in extreme cases, removal of the eye.

Corrugator supercilii: the corrugator supercilii is a small, narrow, pyramidal muscle placed at the medial end of the eyebrow, beneath the frontalis and just above orbicularis oculi. The corrugators draws the eyebrow downward and toward the middle, producing the vertical wrinkles of the forehead. It is the "frowning" muscle and may be regarded as the principal muscle in the expression of suffering. This muscle can be inactivated with Botox as a preventive treatment for some types of migraine or for aesthetic reasons.

Auricular muscles: the auricular muscles are comprised of three (anterior, superior, and posterior) muscles surrounding the auricula or outer ear. In other animals these muscles serve to rotate the auricula to point in the direction of interesting sounds; in most humans all they can manage is a feeble wiggle.

Orbicularis oris: the orbicularis oris muscle is the sphincter muscle around the mouth. It is a complex of muscles in the lips that encircle the mouth and closes the mouth or puckers the lips when it contracts. The depressor labii inferioris helps lower the bottom lip.

Triangularis: the depressor anguli oris or triangularis arises from the oblique line of the mandible where its fibers come together to be inserted by a narrow fasciculus into the angle of the mouth. It is a muscle of facial expression associated with frowning.

Levator labii superioris: the levator labii superioris (or quadratus labii superioris) is a broad sheet muscle that extends from the side of the nose to the zygomatic bone. The levator labii superioris alaeque nasi muscle is, translated from Latin, the "lifter of the upper lip and of the wing of the nose." It has the longest name of any muscle. It dilates the nostril and elevates the upper lip, enabling one to snarl.

Zygomatic major: the zygomatic major is a muscle of facial expression that draws the angle of the mouth superiorly and posteriorly for smiling. The zygomaticus extends from each zygomatic arch (cheekbone) to the corners of the mouth. It raises the corners of the mouth when a person smiles. Dimples may be caused by variations in the structure of this muscle.

Zygomaticus minor: the zygomaticus minor originates from malar bone and continues with orbicularis oculi on the lateral face of the levator labii superioris and then inserts into the outer part of the upper lip. This muscle should not be confused with the zygomaticus major, which inserts into the angle of the mouth. It draws the upper lip backward, upward, and outward and is usually used in making sad facial expressions.

Risorius: the risorius arises in the fascia over the parotid glands and passes horizontally forward superficially to the platysma and inserts into the skin at the angle of the mouth. The risorius retracts the angle of the mouth to produce a smile, albeit an insincere-looking one that does not involve the skin around the eyes. Compare with a real smile, which raises the lips with the action of the zygomaticus major and the zygomaticus minor muscles and causes "crow's feet" around the eyes using the orbicularis oculi muscles.

Caninus: the levator anguli oris (caninus) is the facial muscle of the mouth arising from the canine fossa, immediately below the infraorbital foramen. Its fibers are inserted into the angle of the mouth, intermingling with those of the zygomaticus, the triangularis, and the orbicularis oris. Specifically, the levator anguli oris is innervated by the buccal branches of the facial nerve.

Buccinator: the buccinator is a thin quadrilateral muscle occupying the interval between the maxilla and the mandible at the side of the face. Its purpose is to pull back the angle of the mouth and to flatten the cheek area, which aids in holding the cheek to the teeth during chewing. It aids in whistling and smiling, and in neonates it is used to suckle.

Mentalis: the mentalis is a paired central muscle of the lower lip situated at the tip of the chin. It raises and pushes up the lower lip, causing wrinkling of the chin as in doubt or displeasure. It is sometimes referred to as the "pouting muscle."

Figure 8.4.

Anatomy of the muscles of the facial expressions

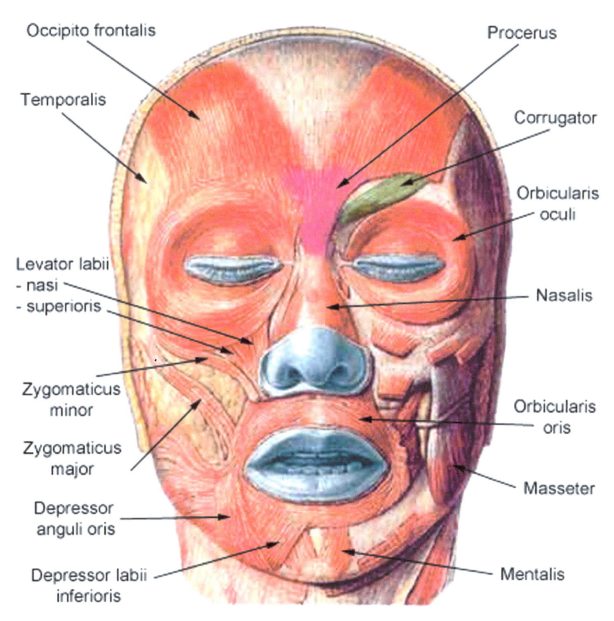

chapter 9

Cosmetic Botulinum Toxin (BOTOX)

INTRODUCTION TO BOTULINUM TOXIN

BOTOX COSMETICS

BOTOX INJECTION SITES

BOTOX INJECTION TECHNIQUES

DOSE OF INJECTIONS

RECONSTITUTION AND STORAGE

GLABELLAR FROWN LINES INJECTION

FOREHEAD LINES AND WRINKLES INJECTION

TEMPORAL EYEBROW LIFT

BOTOX FOR THE REDUCTION OF CROW'S FEET LINES

NOSE-CROSS WRINKLES (BUNNY LINES) INJECTION

BOTOX FOR THE REDUCTION OF NECK CORDS

BOTOX INJECTION TECHNIQUES FOR NECK CORD TREATMENT

BOTOX FOR THE TREATMENT OF HYPERHIDROSIS (EXCESSIVE SWEATING)

STARCH/IODINE SWEAT TEST

ARMPIT INJECTION OF BOTOX FOR HYPERHIDROSIS TREATMENT

THERAPEUTIC BOTOX

BOTOX TREATMENT FOR MIGRAINE

TREATMENT OF MUSCLE SPASMS WITH BOTOX

TREATMENT OF ENLARGED PROSTATES WITH BOTOX

BOTOX SIDE EFFECTS

BOTOX CONTRAINDICATIONS

BOTOX PROS AND CONS

CHAPTER 9

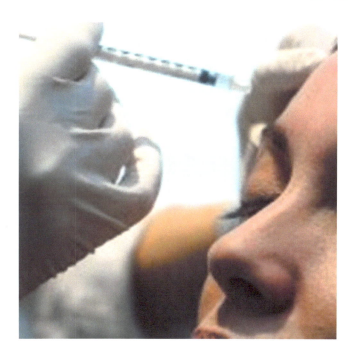

Cosmetic Botulinum Toxin (Botox)

INTRODUCTION TO BOTULINUM TOXIN

Botulinum toxin type A (BTX-A or Botox), widely known by its trade name Botox is used for various cosmetic and medical procedures. Botulinum toxin is a protein produced by the bacteria *Clostridium botulinum*. This bacterial toxin is extremely toxic for the nervous system in its natural form and causes flaccid muscular paralysis. However, as an approved prescription drug by the FDA used in medical settings, injection of sterile, purified, and small doses of Botox has become a routine procedure in medical aesthetics. Botox blocks the nerve impulses and the release of acetylcholine, a neurotransmitter that regulates muscle contraction and, hence, temporarily paralyzes and disables the muscles that are responsible for facial movement.

Botulinum toxin causes selective weakening of muscles by interrupting the nerve signal transmitting from the nerve to the muscle at the neuromuscular junction. Once the muscle does not contract the overlying skin cannot wrinkle and fold. For example, Botox is used to relax the muscles between the eyebrows, across the forehead and neckline, and inactivate the muscles that are involved in wrinkling the skin. The effects can last about four to six months, eliminating the frustrated or angry look in the treated individual when a facial expression is made. Repeated injection leads to longer-lasting results. Given that the treatment only relaxes the muscle underlying the injection site, it fortunately has no effect on other elements of facial expression. In addition, a Botox injection has no effect on the sensory nerves, thus the normal sense of touch and feeling in the treated areas remains unaffected.

COSMETIC BOTOX

American plastic surgeon Dr. Richard Clark originally showed the cosmetic effect of botulinum toxin-A (BTX-A) on wrinkles in 1989. Subsequently, Canadian scientist-clinicians Alastair and Jean Carruthers were the first to publish a study on BTX-A for the treatment of glabellar frown lines in 1992. Once approved by the FDA in 2002, Botox cosmetics have provided an excellent safety track record as an alternative for invasive plastic surgery and facelift. It has now been used in more than seventy countries for cosmetic purposes.

Botox plays a great role in modern medical aesthetics by temporarily eliminating or reducing dynamic wrinkles of the face and neck. The results of Botox cosmetics can last between three to eight months. Therefore, compared to relatively permanent surgical procedures, it has been even more favored by people who consider the reversible effect of Botox therapy if other options are desired at later points in time. Overall, cosmetic Botox meets the criteria of a nonsurgical cosmetic procedures due to effectiveness, safety, simplicity, noninvasivness, minimal discomfort, affordability, and timeliness. Botox has earned its first position among all cosmetic procedures in North America.

Figure 9.1. Botox mechanisms of action

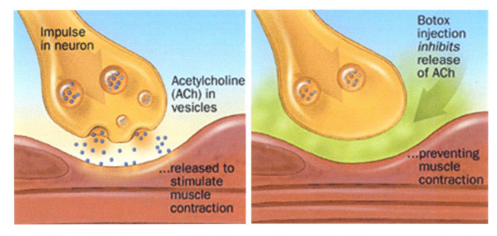

Our brain sends electrical messages to the muscles so that they can contract and move. The electrical message is transmitted to the muscle by a substance called acetylcholine. BTX-A works to block the release of acetylcholine and, as a result, the muscle doesn't receive the message to contract. This means that the muscle spasms stop or are greatly reduced after using the toxin. In cosmetics use, BTX-A temporarily paralyses the muscles responsible for facial expressions and, hence, reduces the wrinkles produced by those expressions.

After cosmetic Botox was initially performed as a treatment for brow lines and wrinkles and glabellar furrows, it was then administered in brow depressor muscles to elevate the brows. Interestingly, Botox relaxes the brow depressor muscles, allowing the eyes a more open, lifted look. Therefore, it can be used to equalize the height of the brows. Subsequently, cosmetic Botox was used to improve horizontal forehead lines and crow's feet wrinkles beside the eyes. In addition, the cosmetic Botox treats vertical lip lines by affecting the orbicularis oris muscle, softens the mouth frown by influencing the depressor anguli oris muscle, and treats the apple dumpling chin by inactivating the mentalis muscle. Furthermore, cosmetic Botox is also commonly applied to treat vertical neck bands resulted from contraction of platysmal muscles.

After a surgical facelift, injection of Botox in the platysma muscle can prevent dragging of the incision line and thus, the wound closure is faster and the healing process does not yield to an obtrusive and visible scar. Cosmetic Botox can also be used in order to reduce the size of scars by providing a relaxed, tension-free healing process and improve the nature and texture of the skin. Cosmetic Botox can be used alone or can be combined with the soft tissue filler treatments or with lasers and other energy-based devices to achieve optimal cosmetic results in the desired areas.

Figure 9.2. Botox

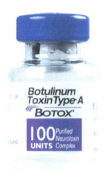

Commercially available botulinum toxin (Botox) from Allergan

BOTOX INJECTION SITES

Botox is most commonly used to smooth out glabellar frown lines (those deep creases between the eyebrows), forehead wrinkles caused by raising the eyebrows, and crow's feet (wrinkles on the lateral aspect of the eyes cause by squinting or smiling). Botox can also used to diminish upper lip wrinkles (smoker's lines around the lips), mouth frown lines, eyebrow frown lines, worry lines, bunny lines on the nose, and the appearance of irregular dimpled skin on the chin. Neckbands or necklace lines that appear on the neck with age can be treated and eliminated with Botox as well.

Performed by experienced cosmetic physicians who are knowledgeable of facial muscle anatomy, Botox injections can be used to enhance the arch shape of the eyebrows, the shape of the mouth by lifting its corners up, and the reduction chin dimpling. Below are most common uses of cosmetics Botox:

- horizontal forehead lines
- vertical lines between the brows
- crow's feet
- brow lowering or brow elevation
- downturning of the mouth
- bunny lines on the side of nose
- vertical upper lip lines
- turkey necklines
- horizontal necklines

- excessive underarm/hand/foot sweating
- essential blepharospasm, hemifacial spasm, facial tics
- torticollis, various focal dystonias
- laryngeal spasms
- tension headache, migraine headaches, and many others
- spastics muscles in cerebral palsy
- back spasms

BOTOX INJECTION TECHNIQUES

The area of injection should be cleansed first with an antiseptic solution. Depending on the patient's comfort level, the procedure can be performed without desensitizing or the skin may be locally anesthetized with a cream and/or ice. However, topical anesthetics are dilators and, therefore, may increase diffusion of Botox to unwanted areas. Botox injections are usually administered with a very small needle, most commonly a 30-gauge tuberculin syringe with a half-inch needle. Thirty units of Botox can be placed into the syringe. The optimal volume of injection is approximately five units of Botox per site into the muscle along the wrinkle.

A new syringe should be used after every five injections. Injections can be made at about 1 cm intervals along the line of the wrinkle. For coarse wrinkles, injections may be made both above and below the wrinkles. Multiple injections of small amounts of toxin create weakness without total paralysis. Regular activities can be resumed after the injections, however, it is recommended that the patient not to lie down or engage in vigorous physical activities over four hours after the injections.

DOSE OF INJECTIONS

The dose of Botox is articulated in mouse-units. One unit is the amount that when injected within the peritoneums of a group of twenty-gram Swiss-Webster mice would have lethal effect on half of the group. The lethal dose for Botox in humans is about 3000 units. However, there is a broad protection range for the use of Botox in humans. For cosmetic purposes, injection of Botox is estimated at about 100 units and for therapeutic treatment is usually about 300–600 units. The toxin can be diluted at a rate of 100 units (one vial) per milliliter (figure). This dilution can be used for dosages greater than 5 units per injection.

For smaller dosages, a vial of 100 units of Botox can be diluted in 2 ml. This provides more dispersal around the injection site, which probably results in a steadier and uniform effect. On the other hand, if side effects such as tearing, ptosis (eyelid drooping), or diplopia (double vision) are a concern, injection with a less diluted toxin (100 units in 0.5 milliliter) may eliminate side effects yet provide a desirable response. The average number of injections per visit may be maintained at about ten shots.

RECONSTITUTION AND STORAGE

Lyophilized Botox must be kept in a freezer at or below -5°C. Once reconstituted, it should be stored at 2–8°C and used within four hours. Commonly, a 100-unit vial is reconstituted in 1 ml of sterile saline. Practically, more concentrated solutions increase the reliability in delivering an accurate unit doses while more dilute solutions lead to greater diffusion of the toxin. The most preferred dilution is dissolving the 100 units of the toxin in 2 ml of saline. This will prepare a solution of 50 units in a 1-ml syringe. Most practitioners discard unused reconstituted Botox after seven days.

GLABELLAR FROWN LINES INJECTION

Glabellar frown lines are the most common treatment area for the cosmetic injection of Botox. To locate the muscles, the patient is asked to frown and scowl. The target muscles may be examined by touching. To achieve acceptable effect, 5 units of toxin can be injected in five sites in muscles that are responsible for making glabellar frown lines for total dose of 25 units. Briefly, the corrugator muscle receives two injections one on each side, the orbicularis oculi and depressor supercilii are injected one site on each side, and the procerus muscle in the midline gets one injection. When injecting the corrugator muscle the needle should be placed above the medial canthus and superciliary arch until bone is felt. The needle then must be withdrawn slightly before inserting the toxin.

Figure 9.3. Glabellar frown lines injection site

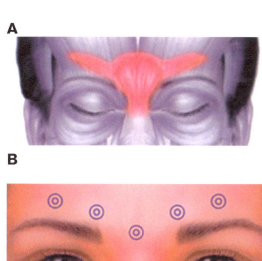

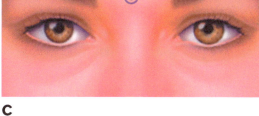

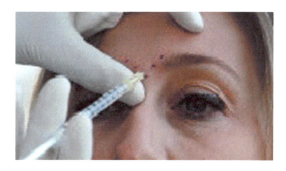

Glabellar frown lines are the most common treatment by Botox procedure. (A) The folds in this area are caused by vertically oriented muscles. (B and C) When treating glabellar frown lines, about five sites are to be administered with the toxin. About 25 units are used for all five sites.

FOREHEAD LINES AND WRINKLES INJECTION

Treatment of horizontal forehead lines with Botox injections is reasonably simple and straightforward. The result usually is very rewarding. A primary injection site about 1 cm above the eyebrow vertical to the medial canthus should be selected first. This procedure includes injection of four sites on each side of the midline using 1–3 units of Botox per site with 1–2 cm distance intervals. Three additional injections laterally and upward to the hairline may be performed. Injections of the upper face and periocular region are usually performed with the patient seated, and the patient is asked to remain upright for 2–3 hours to prevent spread of toxin through the orbital septum.

Figure 9.4. Forehead lines and wrinkles injection sites

A

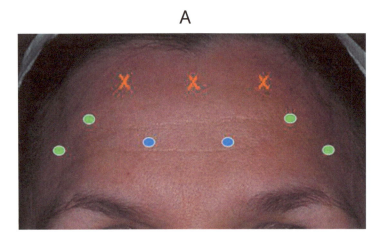

B

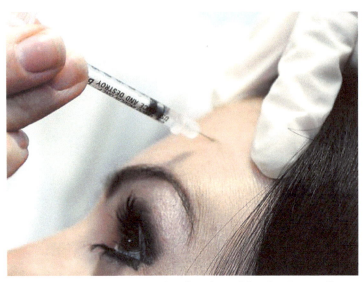

Typical Botox injection spots on the forehead in the frontalis muscles.

TEMPRORAL EYEBROW LIFT

The eyebrow lift is a highly sought procedure among younger and middle-aged women. Aging causes the lateral eyebrow to naturally become ptotic before the medial aspect, resulting in a steady decline of the forehead and brow in the upper third of the face from the hairline to the top of the eyebrows. Injecting the depressor muscles creates a lifting effect alleviating the depressed-looking eyes common in middle age. Temporal brow lifts can be achieved by injections into the lateral brow depressors.

For a 1–5 mm elevation of eyebrow, about 8 units of Botox must be injected into the superolateral portion of the orbicularis oculi muscle below the lateral third of the brow. Injection of the superior and lateral to the orbital rim can minimize the possibility of ptosis. In the illustration below, circles represent the fairly accurate injection zone area. Before the procedure, the natural shape of the eyebrows should be examined for any unevenness that may require correction. Then an eyebrow slope and treatment should be planned accordingly. Figure 9.5 illustrates the ideal brow position for a desirable-looking eyebrow.

Figure 9.5. Ideal brow position

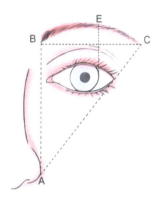

The brow is not a straight line, and it peaks at the outer margin of the iris (point E). The medial and lateral edges of the brow (B and C) are at about the same level. If the medial part of the eyebrow is relatively too high, it give an "exclaming" or "sad" look. On the other hand, when the lateral edge of the brow is relatively too high, it gives the appearance of being mad or angry.

Figure 9.6. Injection site for an eyebrow lift

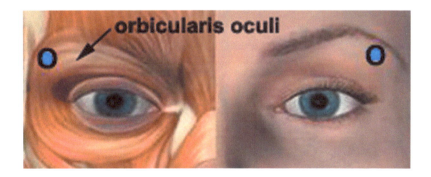

In order to raise the eyebrow, the injection must be performed upward into the orbicularis cculi muscle that draws the eyebrow down. The injection is done slightly under the eyebrow.

The typical appropriate dosage range for Botox treatment of the lateral brow lift is around 5 Botox units per injection point. Typically, success is achieved via precise injections in the superior and lateral aspect of orbicularis oculi, one per side, approximately 0.5 cm above the orbital rim as indicated by blue circles in the illustration (figure 9.6). In summary, a lateral brow lift refers to placing Botox in the outer edge of the eyebrows to create a subtle lifting of this area. This outcome is natural in its appearance because it allows the brows to return to their normal position when the eye muscle isn't contracting and pulling this area down.

Lateral brow lifts are often performed in combination with other upper face procedures. Multiple muscles such as the frontalis, corrugators, procerus, and the orbicularis oculi have an impact on brow position. The usual action of the frontalis is to raise the eyebrows in the expression of surprise, and even higher with fright, and to furrow the forehead with transverse lines with thought. It is crucial that an experienced practitioner performs the procedure as an inaccuracy in the injection may yield to more asymmetrical eyebrows and/or droopy eyelid.

BOTOX FOR THE REDUCTION OF CROW'S FEET LINES

Crow's feet are those little lines on the side of the eyes that can age the appearance far more rapidly than many other skin conditions. Named for their forked appearance, somewhat like a crow's foot, the horizontal lines and wrinkles on the outer aspect of the eyes and eyelids (figure 9.7 C) can give an impression of aging. Since these lines are usually the result of hyperactive muscular activities in this area, they can easily be treated with Botox injections (shown as black dots in figure 9.7 A).

Treatment with Botox relaxes the underlying muscles and results in reduction of these lines and wrinkles. Although it is effective in reducing the facial lines that are due to muscular hyperactivity, treatment is not suitable for static wrinkles caused by photodamage or by muscle laxity in the periorbital area. Treating crow's feet lines requires only very low doses of Botox, usually 15 units into the crow's feet (7.5 units on each side or 2.5 units on each injection site; figure 9.7 B) yields a satisfactory results.

Figure 9.7

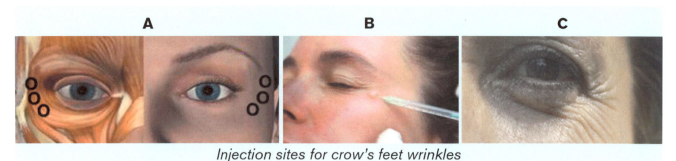

Injection sites for crow's feet wrinkles

NOSE-CROSS WRINKLES (BUNNY LINES) INJECTION

Bunny line wrinkles, which appear on the lateral/dorsal aspects of the nose but which may extend out to the lower eyelid, are present in some people naturally during expression. The contraction of the nasalis muscles is responsible for bunny line wrinkles. Patients should be asked to laugh, sniff, and to squint intensely. Usually, bunny lines become evident when smiling at maximum contraction. Circles in figure 9.8 (A–B) represent the approximate injection zone area for Botox treatment of the nasalis muscle. Bunny lines may be treated alone or in conjunction with the treatment of crow's feet and glabellar lines. Bunny lines are typically treated via two lateral injections totaling 5 to 10 Botox units into the nasalis.

Figure 9.8. Injection sites for bunny line wrinkles
A   **B**

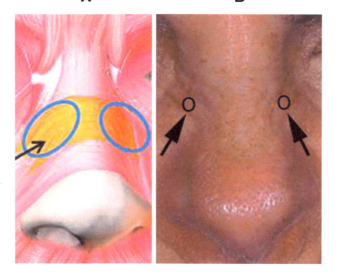

BOTOX FOR THE REDUCTION OF NECK CORDS

Age-related descending drag of the thin muscle (platysma muscle) causes perpendicular fibrous bands known as neck cords. A number of reasons affect aging of the neck, including heredity and weight loss. Inactivating platysma with Botox injections can reduce the neck cord contraction and effectively decrease neck cords, thereby the platysma muscle loses contractile property to form the prominent folds that extend across the vertical length of the neck. A cosmetic physician must diagnose the neck cord and carefully select the right client for the treatment since not all cord-like features in the neck area are due to muscle contraction. Cosmetic Botox injections of the neck are commonly performed for younger clients with strong platysmal bands, older clients who have high risk factor for the surgery, or those who have severe neck skin excess.

Figure 9.9. Age-related neck cords

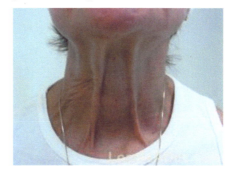

BOTOX INJECTION TECHNIQUES FOR NECK CORD TREATMENT

The area of injection should be cleansed with an antiseptic solution. After skin preparation, the client will be instructed to contract platysma muscle in order to locate the neckbands associated with the contraction. The injection can be performed at 1.0- to 1.5-cm intervals from the jawline to the lower neck. Depending on the thickness of platysmal band, between 3–10 units of Botox should be injected in each injection site. The larger bands can be injected with 20 units each and smaller bands with 5 units each. Most individuals need a total of 50–100 units whereas in some it is necessary to inject as many as 200 units. False injection of the muscles beneath the platysma muscles may cause weakness in the swallowing. Side effects are negligible and may include temporary edema and ecchymosed skin, bruising, muscle tenderness, and mild neck weakness.

Figure 9.10. Neck cord treatment before and after

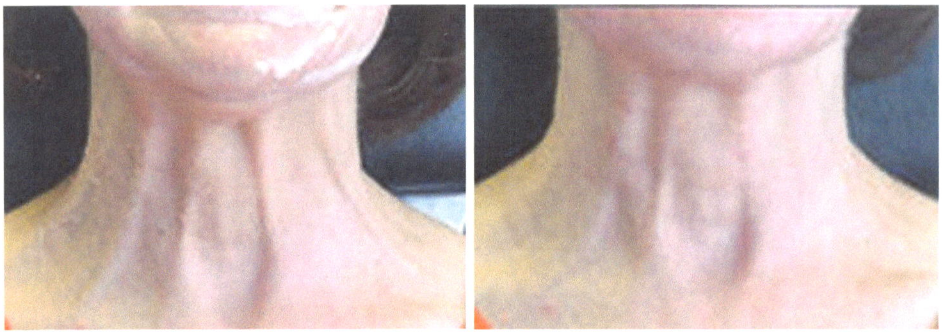

Before   After

Neck cords can be reduced by paralyzing the platysma muscle extended from the jawline to the lower neck with Botox injection. Once relaxed the muscle does not contract to form the prominent folds that run the vertical length of the neck. Not all folds/cords due to muscle contraction, and it is important to carefully select the right client for best treatment possible.

BOTOX FOR TREATMENT OF HYPERHYDROSIS (EXCESSIVE SWEATING)

Hyperhidrosis or excessive production of sweat affects about 1% of the population. It is caused by overactivity of eccrine sweat glands in the skin. Eccrine sweat glands are concentrated throughout the skin in the palms, soles, and under the armpits (axillae). Eccrine sweat evaporates on the surface of the skin and affects a transfer of heat, mainly by direct transmission from the vascular supply to the skin, thereby maintaining body temperature in the event of external heat or increase in physical activity. Eccrine glands are surrounded by myoepithelial cells, which contract upon stimulation from the sympathetic nerves that utilize acetylcholine as their neurochemical transmitter at the nerve endings.

Higher cortical functions in the brain during anxiety and stress together with thermal stress induced by heat or exercise results in the direct stimulation of the glands.

Botox reduces hyperhidrosis by inactivating the contractile properties of myoepithelial cells, thereby reducing the discharge of sweat. In addition, Botox is used to treat excessive sweating of the forehead, scalp, underarms, palms, and feet. A significant reduction more the 80% in sweating within a week can be achieved after the treatment with Botox in the affected areas. In most cases, sweating diminishes substantially within 48 hours and results can last from four to eighteen months.

The procedure is quite simple. A small volume of Botox is injected into the affected area through a very fine needle. The needle is placed just under the skin. Multiple injections are recommended based on the assessment of the area and the condition to be treated. In order to assess the appropriate dosage of Botox to treat hyperhidrosis, a Minor's starch/iodine test is administered to the affected area, which makes the area of sweating visible and determines the severity of the sweating. Usually, men require higher doses than do women.

Figure 9.11. Hyperhidrosis

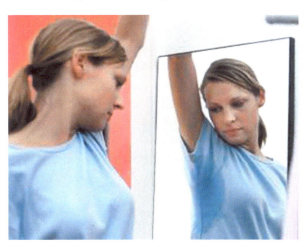

Some individuals sweat in excess, causing problems with school, work, and social situations. Hyperhidrosis affects both males and females and can start at any age. It is often a severe and emotionally distressing problem for people with the condition.

STARCH/IODINE SWEAT TEST

In a Minor test, or starch/iodine sweat test, a 2% iodine solution is applied to the area of interest and allowed to dry. Starch in powder form (corn starch) is then brushed on the area. In areas of sweat, the light brown iodine color turns dark purple as an iodine-starch complex forms in the liquid medium. The worst affected area can be visualized and marked, and photography of the involved area allows for documentation and follow-up comparison after treatment.

Figure 9.12: Starch/iodine sweat test

(1) Iodine is applied to the treatment area. (2) When the area is dry, the starch indicator is applied to the treatment area and left for up to fifteen minutes. (3) The perspiration turns the powder black and indicates the area that needs treating. (4) The area requiring treatment is identified and marked.

Images adobted from caci Medispa Hyperhidrosis Clinic http://nosweat.co.nz/

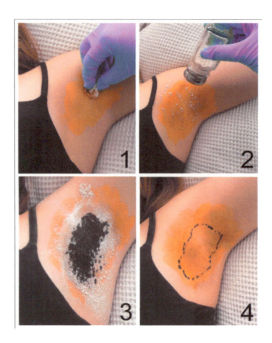

Figure 9.13. Botox injection in armpit for the treatment of excessive sweating

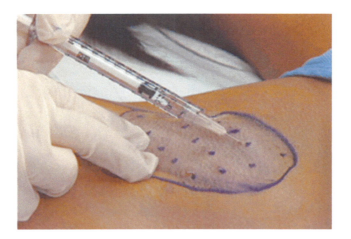

During the procedure, a very fine needle is used to inject small amounts of Botox just under the skin near the sweat glands responsible for excessive perspiration. Multiple injections are given based on the assessment of the area that needs to be treated. To ease discomfort, physicians may use one or more of a number of anesthetic techniques such as painkilling creams, nerve blocks, ice, or vibrations.

AXILLAE INJECTION OF BOTOX FOR HYPERHIRDROSIS TREATMENT

Minimal required dose of Botox is 100 units per underarm. The expected remission period ranges between four and twelve months. Also, a temporary muscle weakness or relaxation following the injections may occur in less than 20% of the patients and may last an average of three weeks. The effect of this treatment is temporary and lasts only for few months, and thus, the treatment has to be repeated two to three times every year. The use of Botox for the treatment of hyperhidrosis is most effective when performed by a physician who has received special training and who has experience with the procedure. Botox injections can be administered in a physician's office, require relatively little time, and do not confine work or leisure activity apart from abstaining from rigorous exercise or the use of a sauna on the day of the injections.

THERAPEUTIC BOTOX

Therapeutic Botox is a safe, effective treatment for many medical conditions and is used in children as young as two. For example, therapeutic Botox can treat muscle spasms, temporomandibular joint disorder, enlarged prostates, excessive perspiration, migraine and other headaches, and neck pain from muscle tension. Medical Botox treatments are often covered by extended-health benefit plans when prescribed by a medical doctor to treat these conditions.

BOTOX TREATMENT FOR MIGRAINE

Botox treatment is used to alleviate the migraine headache, tension headache, temporomandibular joint pain, bruxism, postherpetic neuralgia, and involuntary teeth grinding. Botox is also very useful for patients with chronic soft tissue pain in their heads and necks. Botox is injected into the forehead, neck, and shoulders where patients are experiencing pain and tension. The botulinum toxin is thought to eliminate migraines by reducing muscle tension and thus creating less strain on the nervous system. When injecting Botox for migraines, the treatment is done symmetrically in the facial area. The muscles that are involved in migraine headache and need to be treated with Botox injections are the suboccipital musculature (muscles at the back of the neck), the trapezius, the rhomboids, and the internal pterygoids inside the mouth.

TREATMENT OF MUSCLE SPASMS WITH BOTOX

Spontaneous muscle contractions are known as muscle spasms or muscle spasticity. Muscle spasms are general symptoms of some pathological conditions such as multiple sclerosis and cerebral palsy. A stroke or a spinal cord injury can also develop severe spasticity. Muscle spasms may result in aggravated muscle pains, joint complications, muscle shortening, limb movement, and walking problems.

Once injected in the muscle, the botulinum toxin inhibits cholinergic sensory receptors and temporarily paralyzes or inactivates the muscles, thus eliminating involuntary muscle contractions. Currently, the FDA has approved Botox for muscle spasms in the wrists, fingers, and elbows. Injecting Botox to treat muscle spasms in the upper limbs or legs has not yet been fully tested.

TREATMENT OF ENLARGED PROSTRATES WITH BOTOX

Enlarged prostates are very common in men over the age of sixty, with high frequency. One of the most common symptoms of an enlarged prostate is multiple urination or difficulty urinating. While there are certainly other medical treatments for an enlarged prostate, many of them can lead to sexual side effects, including impotence. Evidence indicates that administering Botox to men who had an enlarged prostate actually relieved symptoms for up to a year after the procedure. Scientifically, it has been shown that Botox injection leads to programmed cell death or, through a process called apoptosis, decreases the size of the prostate gland by reducing of the live cells.

The smaller prostate gland improves the urinary flow and helps decrease the residual urine left in the bladder. In addition to the reduction of cells, the Botox injection paralyzes the prostate gland and contributes to preventing further prostate enlargement. Fortunately, there have been no reports of side effects from Botox injection to the prostate. The results can be seen within two weeks of the initial injection, and long-term results are promising.

BOTOX SIDE EFFECTS

There is no permanent side effect known for Botox therapy for facial wrinkles. The side effects seen following Botox injection are transient and usually negligible. However, some patients may complain about a light pain associated with needle injection sites, minor bruising, itchiness over the injection site, minimal skin redness, and headache. Also, there is a small risk of getting a transient eyelid droop if the injected drug moves into the muscles responsible for elevating the eyelids. This is seen in less than 1% of patients receiving Botox therapy and can be treated with administration of eye drops such as 0.5%-Iodipine once or twice a day for up to a week.

BOTOX CONTRAINDICATIONS

People with the following complications are not the best candidate for Botox therapy: those with severe neuromuscular diseases like myasthenia gravis, Eaton-Lambert syndrome, severe multiple sclerosis, active shingles of the face (herpes zoster), and cold sores (herpes simplex). In addition, Botox injection is not recommended for individuals with a history of severe migraines after Botox cosmetic injections, pregnant women, and women who are breastfeeding.

Other contraindications include prior allergic reaction, injection into areas of infection or inflammation, and patients with diseases of the neuromuscular junction such as myasthenia gravis. Some medications decrease neuromuscular transmission and generally should be avoided in patients treated with Botox. These include aminoglycosides, penicillamine, quinine, and calcium channel blockers.

BOTOX PROS AND CONS

Before going through the procedure, one should know what Botox can and can't do and what the disadvantages might be. Botox is a trade name of botulinum toxin, the base cause of botulism. It is sometimes fatal food poisoning. However, in small quantities Botox only interrupts nerve impulses to muscles in the face and temporarily paralyzes muscles responsible for facial expression, which are often manifested as wrinkles and folds in the face. The FDA has approved Botox for the removal of certain wrinkles.

Fortunately, Botox is substantially diluted so that serious side effects like allergic reactions are uncommon. If the injector makes a mistake—for example, in the areas around eyes—in most cases the worst consequence is losing the ability to raise the eyelids all the way. A mistaken injection around the mouth may result in salivating. Regardless, even a perfectly performed procedure has consequences. Depending on which wrinkles are being treated, the client might not be able to frown or raise his/her eyebrows or narrow the eyes. Fortunately, if there are some unwanted results, Botox wears off after a few months. However, if satisfied with the results, one has to go back every six months at up to several hundred dollars per treatment.

Botox injections must be performed by a trained professional. The reality is that Botox is not a cure for wrinkles; rather, it deters them for few months. In some cases, if you are not a good candidate for the treatment, Botox can actually make you look worse. Botox products are designed for therapeutic uses as well. Initially Botox was used for strictly medical purposes, such as suppressing the unnatural muscle spasms, etc. Some symptoms of neurological conditions can be improved with Botox. A Botox injection is also an effective treatment for excess armpits sweating.

Unfortunately, many individuals have taken to injecting themselves and friends with Botox on their own. This is strongly not recommended. The risk of developing an allergy to Botox is not too high, and even if your skin does adversely react to it, the consequences will not be hard to manage. When the procedure is done by a professional practitioner, the only side effects that might occur are nausea, temporary headaches, swelling, bruising, and pain. Muscle weakness that might limit facial movement is another side effect that can occur and might often be accompanied by flu-like symptoms.

chapter 10

Dermal Fillers

INTRODUCTION TO DERMAL FILLERS

COLLAGEN'S MOLECULAR STRUCTURE

SKIN AND COLLAGEN

THE PROCESS OF COLLAGEN FIBRILLOGENESIS

HYALURONIC ACID (HA)

INJECTABLE DERMAL FILLERS

MOST COMMON INJECTABLE DERMAL FILLERS

RESTYLANE

TEOSYAL

JUVEDERM

RADIESSE

EVOLENCE

ARTESENSE

SCULPTRA

MACROLANE

MACROLANE AND NONSURGICAL BREAST AUGMENTATION

BIO-ALCAMID

SILICONE OIL

FIBRIN-PLATELET FILLS (SELPHYL)

PLATELET-RICH PLASMA THERAPY

DERMAL FILLER INJECTION TECHNIQUES

TYPICAL SITES OF INJECTION

NONSURGICAL RHINOPLASTY (NOSE JOB)

INJECTABLES: RISKS AND SIDE EFFECTS

DERMAL FILLER PREOPERATIONAL CHECKLIST

CHAPTER 10

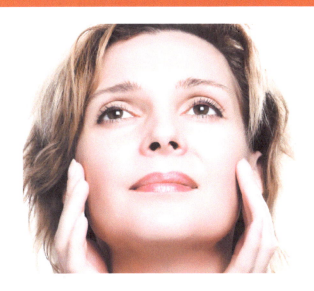

Dermal Fillers

INTRODUCTION TO DERMAL FILLERS

The simplest, least expensive method and ongoing solution for facial contouring can be achieved by temporary injectable substances known as dermal fillers. Over the past several years, a variety of fat-, silicone-, collagen- and hyaluronic acid–based fillers have been used in the medical aesthetics practices. Soft-tissue fillers are the materials that are placed into deeper layers of the skin to correct various facial lines, folds, and wrinkles. The injection of fillers can be done in an office setting with or without a local anesthesia. Therefore, easy application of natural products in cosmetic fillers, minimal complications and side effects, reasonable price, and lower downtime as opposed to traditional cosmetic surgery have contributed to increasing popularity of these products.

Injection of cosmetic fillers has been considered as the third most popular cosmetic procedure in North America. Along with treating wrinkles and skin texture, replacing volume creates a foundation beneath the surface to support the skin and diminishes the look of the lines and wrinkles that come with aging. For example, replacing the natural fat pad of the cheek can create a small lift and will diminish the depth of the nasolabial fold. Among all injectable fillers, collagen- and hyaluronic acid–based products have gained popularity in the medical cosmetics field and the industry for skin rejuvenation.

Most of the cosmetic filler products contain hyaluronic acid as the ground substance, which hydrates the skin, allowing it to appear smoother and more radiant. Clinical studies have shown that hyaluronic acid also promotes the wound-healing process to happen more quickly and can reduce the appearance of both old and new scars. In this chapter, the most common cosmetic dermal fillers and their ground substances, doses, usages, storage methods, and injection methods are discussed in detail.

MOLECULAR STRUCTURE OF COLLAGEN

A molecule of collagen is composed of three main amino acids called lysine, proline, and hydroxyproline. Vitamin C is required in the enzymatic processes of the posttranslational modification of collagen synthesis; thus, vitamin C deficiencies can cause some abnormalities such as loss of teeth, scurvy, and easy bruising. Bruising of skin in collagen deficiency is due to a reduction in the strength of connective tissue.

Poor internal health, poor diet, heredity, or environmental stresses (such as sun's harmful radiation) can cause loss of collagen or prevent the formation of enough collagen that may affect the skin appearance. Orally taken collagen supplements are not effective in restoring collagen loss in the body simply because collagen is just a protein that will be broken down into amino acids in the stomach. Unfortunately, collagen in topical skin care products and makeup cannot be absorbed entirely into the body through the skin. Therefore, a careful combination of external and internal factors must be considered to prevent collagen deficiencies and skin aging.

SKIN AND COLLAGEN

Collagen is the major insoluble fibrous protein in the extracellular matrix of bones, tendons, and skin. Being close to a fourth of all the protein in our body and the main protein of connective tissue, collagen is the most abundant protein in mammals. Connective tissue is considered a glue that holds the body together. It consists of ground substances, namely proteoglycans and hyaluronic acid. The ground substances occupy spaces between the cells and fibers of connective tissues.

Collagen is also the main component of the cornea in a transparent form. Collagen has strong tensile strength and is responsible for skin elasticity. It is also the main constituent of ligaments and tendons. Degradation and/or abnormalities in collagen synthesis often result in skin fragility, wrinkles, and folds.

THE PROCESS OF COLLAGEN FIBRILLOGENSIS

Fibroblasts are the major cell type of the dermis that produce fibrillar form of collagen, and elastic fibers. Procollagen, or the molecular preform of collagen, is composed of a triple helix of polypeptide chains (glycine-proline-hydroxyproline repeating in triplets) containing globular C and N termini. Once N and C ends are cleaved by procollagen peptidase, the molecular collagen is cross-linked together and forms fibrils. Collagen fibrils are packed together and form collagen fibers.

Assembly of several collagen fibers together results in formation of collagen fiber bundles. These tightly cross-linked collagen fibers provide tensile strength and resistance to shear and other mechanical forces. There are over twenty types of collagen in the body. However, fibrillar collagen types I and III are abundantly present in the skin. Elastic fibers play a critical role by resisting deformational changes and returning the skin to its original resting shape.

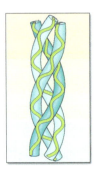

Figure 10.1: Molecular Shape of Collagen

The actual collagen molecule is a "triple helix" or three strands nested together to look a bit like an extremely fine rope. This triple helix is directly responsible for natural gut's elasticity and ability to act like a shock absorber.

Figure 10.2. Collagen fiber structure

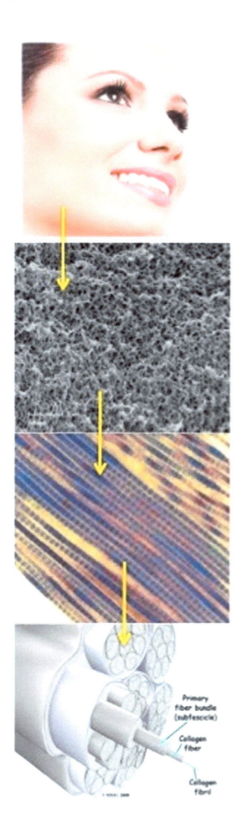

HYALURONIC ACID (HA)

Hyaluronic acid (HA) is a polysaccharide that is naturally found in many tissues of the body, such as in the skin's connective tissue and in cartilage. Particularly, hyaluronan is an important component of articular cartilage, where it is present as a coat around the cells (the chondrocytes). HA maintains the strength and flexibility of cartilage and joints and promotes the joint-lubricating synovial fluid. Without adequate amounts of HA, the joints will become fragile and deteriorated.

HA has a strong affinity to bind to water particles. One of the most important properties of HA is the facilitation of water retention in other bodily tissues. Thereby it keeps moisture into the extracellular matrix. Hyaluronan forms large highly negatively-charged aggregates when it binds to aggrecan, a proteoglycan (sugar-bond protein), in the presence of link protein. These aggregates absorb water and are responsible for the flexibility of cartilage and its resistance to compression.

Hyaluronan is also a major component of skin, where it is involved in tissue repair. When skin is excessively exposed to UVB rays, it becomes inflamed, and the cells in the dermis stop producing as much hyaluronan and increase the rate of its degradation. Hyaluronan also contributes to tissue hydrodynamics and the movement and proliferation of cells, and it participates in a number of cell-surface receptor interactions.

In 2003, the FDA approved hyaluronan injections for filling soft tissue defects such as facial wrinkles. There have been no serious side effects associated with HA, although some people may find that their skin is irritated at the injection site. HA forms a viscous fluid with exceptional lubricating properties necessary for vital functions of many parts of the human body, including skin, heart valves, aqueous/vitreous humor of the eye, joints, and synovial fluid. HA is considered as the secret of all young, smooth skins. Skin contains over 50% of the total HA in the body of an adult. Therefore, it is a basic building block of the dermis that binds water and is responsible for the skin volume. The amount of skin HA decreases with aging. Consequently, aging results in reduced dermal hydration and increased skin wrinkling.

Figure 10.3

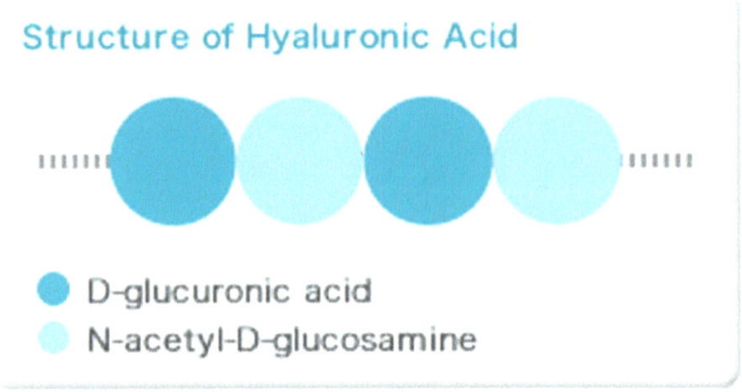

Structure of Hyaluronic Acid

- D-glucuronic acid
- N-acetyl-D-glucosamine

Hyaluronic acid is a linear polysaccharide formed by alternating D-glucuronic acid and N-acetyl-D-glucosamine units. It is found in synovial fluid, the hyaloids of eyes, the skin, the umbilical cords of mammals, and also in cockscombs.

INJECTABLE DERMAL FILLERS

Several companies manufacture long-lasting hyaluronic acid products under different brand names. In recent years, hyaluronic acid–derived products such as Restylane, Hylaform, Juvederm, or Teosyal have gained tremendous popularity and are considered the most common and effective space-filling substances in the human body, particularly for facial skin enhancement.

Macrolane is produced from stabilized nonanimal hyaluronic acid. Many physicians see advantages in using Macrolane for breast shaping as opposed to more invasive techniques. These derma fillers simply work by attracting water from the surrounding tissue due to the action of hyaluronic acid. Thus, conserving dermal hyaluronic acid is an important goal of a successful skin rejuvenation program that helps to achieve younger-looking skin.

Hyaluronic acid products generally last for eight to twelve months, with some variation between each individual a new generation of modified collagen-based fillers or calcium hydroxylapatite offers a choice that lasts long, up to two years. Sculptra is a novel filler containing poly-L-lactic acid, a substance that restores that lost volume of face by stimulating the growth of new collagen.

Sculptra is intended as an implant in cases of severe volume loss and massive fat atrophy. The modern long-lasting collagen-based fillers like Evolence and Evolence Breeze are produced with no human-derived components and have successfully provided satisfactory results for the clients. Injection of dermal fillers is ideally combined with botulinum toxin treatment, which is used for wrinkles caused by too much muscle tone. Ideally, antiaging skin protocols may include filler agents, use of Botox, and skin collagen enhancement.

MOST COMMON INJECTABLE DERMAL FILLERS

Dermal fillers are divided into two groups of large-volume and small-volume injectables. The latter groups, the most common fillers that are used in many medical spa clinics, are three-dimensional volume fillers that correct facial wrinkles, lines, or depressions. The effect is temporary and short-lasting, spanning approximately three to six months. Short-lasting injectables are desirable for clients who want to learn about the effect before considering a prolonged, lasting injectable procedure, for those who are unsure about the correction and want to experience it first, and for those who want an immediate treatment before a social occasion.

Severe facial volume loss due to aging, trauma, and disease can be treated with large-volume injectable fillers. They can be used instead of fat transfers, nasal dorsal implants, chin implants, midface implants, and cheekbone implants, or if large area of facial structures need to be corrected. As little as 2 and as much as 30 ml of the product can be injected at once, and the desired correction can be distinguished faster.

The most common injectable fillers used in medical aesthetic clinics include all hyaluronic acid-based fillers such as Restylane, Perlane Teosyal, and Juvederm. These products are made of a stabilized hyaluronic acid that is produced biosynthetically. High-viscosity versions of Teosyal and Juvederm are usually used for clients requesting a long-lasting treatment. Both Teosyal and Juvederm are very dense, and the implant very slowly disintegrates in the skin after the injection.

Cross-linking of the molecules of hyaluronic acid is used to increase density of the filler and to facilitate its longevity. A Radiesse injection is greatly efficient for nasolabial fold correction while Evolence and Evolence Breeze work great for lips and skin folds. The modern collagen-based fillers like Evolence and Evolence Breeze are produced with no human-derived components. The fillers are bio-compatible and require no allergic reaction assessment. Health Canada and the FDA has approved use of Evolence.

Figure10.4. Facial volume loss

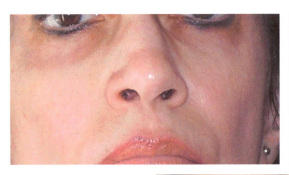
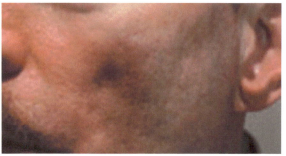
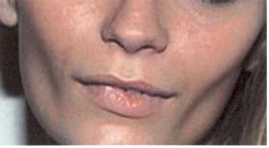

Severe facial volume loss can be corrected by long-lasting dermal filler by injecting of as little as 2 and as much as 30 ml of the product.

RESTYLANE

Restylane is a medium-viscosity hyaluronic filler used primarily for lip enhancement and deeper lines, for the nose bridge, and for the brows. It is a biodegradable nonanimal hyaluronic acid–based filler. In the form of a crystal-clear gel, Restylane injected into the skin efficiently lifts the lips, wrinkles, or folds. In contrast to other biodegradable implants, Restylane is safe to use without pretesting since it is not of animal origin and has no risk of allergic reactions.

Upon injection, Restylane interacts with endogenous hyaluronic acid to build up volume under the skin, where it is intended to work. Effect of Restylane treatment depends on the structure of the skin, lifestyle, and age of the client. Compared to permanent implants, the effect of Restylane remains six to nine months after treatment. Given the fact that face volume is constantly changing and beauty is best maintained by periodically evaluating the need for further implants, and being a temporary filler, treatment with Restylane leaves further options and alternatives when the effect has faded out.

Restylane gel is injected into the skin in tiny amounts with a very fine needle. The result is instantaneous and long-lasting. However, many clients may find it a painful experience with lip injections due to numerous sensory nerve endings in the lips and/or inadequate local anesthetic agents. Perlane, another member of this group of fillers, is structurally manufactured in larger fragments and is intended to be used for filling larger voids and providing more lift to the tissue. Perlane is a higher viscosity hyaluronic acid filler used for deeper folds on the face, like the nasolabial folds. It is used to lift the cheeks and correct nasal defects. Macrolane is most viscous and chunky in the Restylane group. Macrolane has been used in Europe for temporary breast augmentation and filling larger defects.

Figure 10.6. Lip enhancement

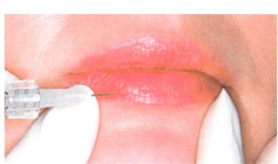

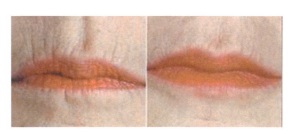

Lip enhancement by Restylane. Restylane procedurea have provided delicate improvement in definition and contouring with a satisfying outcome, as seen immediately following the treatment.

TEOSYAL

Teosyal is a hyaluronic acid—derived injectable used for filling facial lines and wrinkles, such as laughter lines around the eyes and the smoker lines or perioral lines above the top lip. It is also used for the enhancement of lips and for correcting small facial scars and minor imperfections. Teosyal is the most concentrated form of hyaluronic acid available that can be used for cheek augmentation for filling nasolabial (nose to mouth) lines and correction of oral commissures (corners of mouth).

The effect of Teosyal usually lasts eight to twelve months, however, it may last four to six months for lip enhancement depending on age, skin type, the area treated, the volume injected, and the technique used for the procedure. Teosyal has been designed to provide a long-lasting injectable by an extensive cross-linking process which generates a dense network between the hyaluronic acid molecules. The synthesized larger molecules are more resilient to disintegration once injected.

JUVEDERM

Juvederm is made of cross-linked hyaluronic acid chains formulated to be a very soft, pliant, and long-lasting filler gel. Juvederm has been approved by the FDA and Health Canada and widely used in cosmetics corrections. Typical results of treatment are immediate and last from eight to twelve months. Juvederm is suitable for softening lines and wrinkles around the mouth, nose, chin, and forehead. It is best used in the mid to deep dermis for the correction of moderate to severe facial wrinkles. It can also be used to augment lips and fill in acne scars. Juvederm is usually applicable for volumizing the face in areas of fat loss, such as in the brows, forehead, zygomatic area, malar area, nasolabial folds, and melomental folds (marionette lines).

Juvederm can be used to recontour the chin and the lower face. Compared to other injectable fillers, Juvederm is generally well tolerated in clients with different backgrounds. Juvederm Ultra is a medium-viscosity hyaluronic filler used primarily for lip enhancement and deeper lines. Juvederm Ultra is available with lidocaine—the addition of lidocaine to the filler results in a much more comfortable injection experience for the clients.

Juvederm Ultra Plus is a higher-viscosity hyaluronic acid filler used for deeper folds on the face, like in the nasolabial folds. It provides more "lift" than Juvederm Ultra and is also available with lidocaine for increased comfort. Unfortunately, a small minority of clients may manifest small bruise following Juvederm injection. Voluma is a hyaluronic acid soft-tissue filler in the Juvederm family. As the name suggests, it is applied to replace volume in the tissues of the face that have been lost through aging in order to restore a more youthful appearance.

Figure 10.7

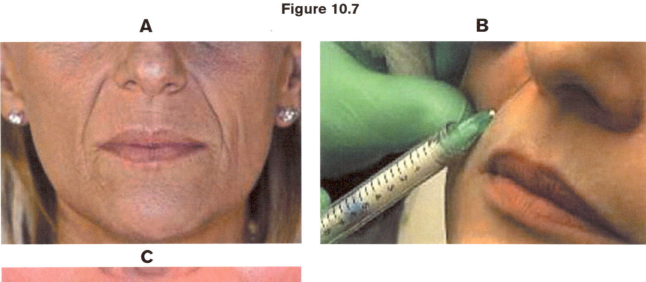
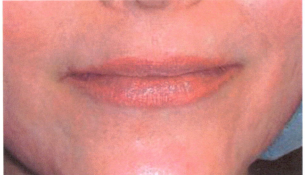

Representative images showing Juvederm injection for reducing nasolabial folds (A–B) also called smile lines and wrinkles/laugh lines. Representative image after the treatment (C).

RADIESSE

Radiesse is a FDA-approved injectable material that is available for aesthetic purposes. It is recommended for lip enhancement and wrinkles and line improvement. It can be used for the correction of nasolabial folds, marionette lines, cheek augmentation, chin augmentation, jawline contouring, mental crease augmentation (chin groove), nasal defects, and hands. Radiesse is made up of microscopic calcium particles, namely hydroxylapatite that is suspended in a carboxymethyl cellulose gel. It is designed with the same mineral component as bone and teeth and, therefore, does not require an allergy test.

The calcium microspheres in Radiesse form a scaffold to support and stimulate the growth of collagen at the site of injection. Over time, the calcium-based microspheres gradually break down and are safely and naturally absorbed by the body. Hydroxylapatite is also implicated in dental reconstruction, bone growth, and vocal cord injections. Radiesse has been proven to be safe and compatible with the body. Radiesse is one of the most long-lasting injectable fillers that lasts from two to five years. Typically, a client who has never had lips augmentation before might choose something less permanent, such as Juvederm or Restylane, if reconsideration of treatment or permanent results is a concern.

EVOLENCE

Evolence is a Health Canada–approved, triple-chain, cross-linked, porcine collagen–based filler composed of a stable collagen compound that lasts about up to twelve months postinjection. It is preferred for use in lip augmentation because of the natural and long-lasting look that can be achieved with minimal swelling at the time of injection. In addition, Evolence can be used to boost up the malor and zygomatic area, nasolabial and melomental folds and to reflate the lower facial margins, including the chin.

When injecting Evolence, it is important to massage the substance immediately because it does tend to set in the place where it has been injected rather quickly. Evolence Breeze is also a Health Canada–approved, triple-chain, cross-linked, porcine collagen filler, but its effect is milder than Evolence, lasting six to nine months. Evolence Breeze is usually injected in areas where a lighter treatment is preferred, such as in the lips or in the nasojugal folds (under the eye hollows).

Figure 10.8. Cheek augmentation

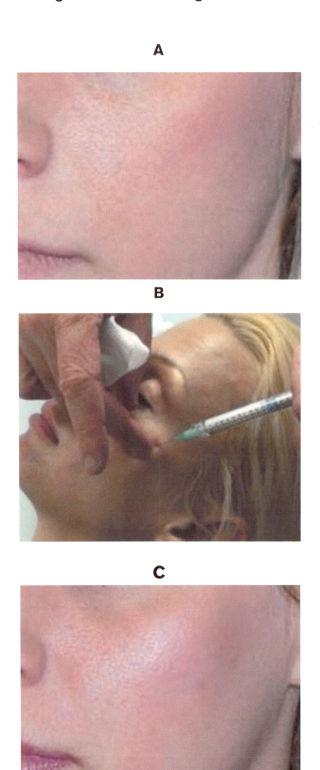

Representative images for cheek augmentation by Radiesse: (A) before, (B) injection to the cheeks, (C) after

ARTESENSE

ArteSense is comprised of small particles called polymethylmethacrylate (PMMA), which are floating in a collagen solution with a local anesthetic. These tiny microbeads are thirty-two to forty micrometers in size, four to five times larger than the size of a red blood cell and well tolerated by human tissue. PMMA has been considered as glue in artificial hip prostheses for many years, with no tendency of rejection. Within ten to twelve weeks postinjection, new collagen will be formed around the microspheres, and the correction of wrinkles or enhancement of desired area can be seen. ArteSense, also known as Artecoll, is a distinctive, long-term, and semi-permanent injectable filler that has been highlighted among medical aesthetics practitioners for its satisfying effect.

Since it is the body's own collagen that is formed at the site of injection, treatment with ArteSense gives up to three to five years of correction results. Deep folds and wrinkles are easily treated with the correct amount of dermal fillers. The degree of correction depends on the client's genetics, physical characteristics, and desire on the volume of filler used. Due to the very long-lasting effect of ArteSense, a consultation with cosmetic physician is necessary to determine the type and volume of correction required. It takes from three to five injections of Artecoll to provide the desired effect.

As the interval between injections is a minimum of two months, the correction may take a year. A skin test is not required prior to starting the injections. Contraindications to the use of ArteSense may be due to a known allergy to the local anesthetic, collagen, or bovine products. Reactions to this product are very uncommon, and if it does occur, treatment with cortisone is recommended to reduce the problem.

Figure 10.9

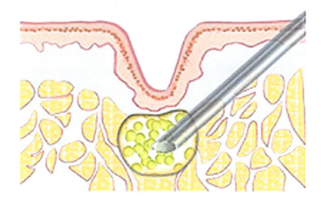

ArteSense is a long-lasting injectable. The gel consists of natural atelocollagen and coated polymethylmetacrylate (PMMA) microbeads and is used for the lasting correction of lines and wrinkles.

SCULPTRA

Originally approved as a filler material for HIV/AIDS patients who had developed significant facial volume reduction, Sculptra is now widely used not only for HIV patients, but also for cosmetic benefits in the general aging population. Sculptra is a novel filler containing poly-L-lactic acid, a substance that restores the lost volume of the face by stimulating growth of new collagen. It is a biocompatible and biodegradable injectable material that naturally stimulates the body to produce its own collagen. Lactic acid is a naturally occurring compound in our body; therefore, a skin reaction test is not required. Polylactic acid is derived from fruit acids. When the micro particles of polylactic acid are deposited under the skin, they begin to stimulate collagen production as they are slowly broken down by the body. A natural and soft increase in dermal thickness begins to take place within several weeks of injection.

Sculptra is especially beneficial for those with thin skin. It is recommended for clients with severe volume loss, well-developed wrinkles, and massive fat atrophy in both the lower and upper face, leading to increased skin thickness, slight and gradual facial volume enhancement, and less pronounced wrinkles and folds. The filling effect of Sculptra can last up to two to three years. As Sculptra is not conventional filler but a collagen modulator, the outcomes will come very gradually. Therefore, the effects may not be seen immediately after injection. However, the results are reported to be very satisfying.

Once Sculptra is injected, the treatment may appear to be immediate. In fact, this is swelling from the injections of the diluents used to reconstitute the product. Within a few days, this initial swelling goes down and the water is absorbed by the body, Repeated treatments sessions provide more opportunity to see the full benefit. The number of treatments may vary from one to four times, depending on the amount of corrections that are desired and the quantity of material used at each treatment session. Over the course of four to six weeks, there is a gradual filling in the hollows, the indentations, and the skin creases, restoring youthful appearance in the facial area that are injected. The improvements typically last several years, and the procedure can be repeated as needed for maintenance.

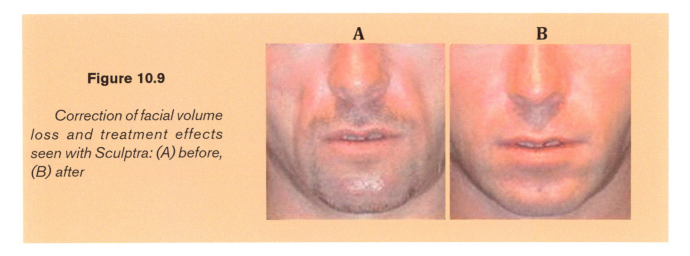

Figure 10.9

Correction of facial volume loss and treatment effects seen with Sculptra: (A) before, (B) after

MACROLANE

Macrolane is a more recent dermal filler that has been used for nonsurgical body shaping. It can be used for large-volume restoration and the shaping of body surfaces, such as in calves and buttocks. Macrolane evens out discrepancies in the skin surface like, for example, those caused by liposuction. Macrolane is mainly desirable for nonsurgical breast augmentation.

Starting in 2008, Macrolane was used for breast shaping in women who have asymmetry, loss of volume as a result of breast feeding or weight loss, or underdeveloped breasts. Macrolane can increase the breast volume by a cup size without the need for surgery. The breast shaping by Macrolane may last for twelve to eighteen months. Top-ups would be required to retain the shape. Macrolane can also smooth up inconsistency in the skin surface like, for example, those caused by liposuction and surgical scars.

MACROLANE AND NONSURGICAL BREAST AUGMENTATION

The risks associated with surgery are major reasons that stop women who consider having breast augmentation. Breast reshaping is the second most wanted body reshaping. Breast implants are highly popular as they may increase self-esteem, confidence, and attractiveness. Fortunately, there is a nonsurgical innovation known as Macrolane injections—introduced initially in Britain—that can increase breast size up to one or one and a half cup sizes. This procedure has attracted many women into considering it over breast implants.

Another advantage of Macrolane is that, unlike traditional surgery, the client can decide for the volume of injection throughout the procedure. In addition, Macrolane is safe because it is a hyaluronic acid–based substance that is naturally exists within the body; therefore, the risk of rejection is none. Finally, the procedure is fast, painless, and without requirement for the recovery. General anesthesia is not required for Macrolane injection. However, local anesthetics may be necessary. The procedure needs minimal time away from work or afterwork activities, but it can be costly and high-maintenance.

Macrolane injection must be performed each year with nearly half the originally injected volume. Generally, 200 ml of Macrolane injection is required for each breast in the first treatment, followed by a 100-ml top-up after twelve months. It is important to monitor that the implant will not adversely affect the efficiency of future mammograms, as well as the breast tissue itself.

Fortunately, to date, studies on mammography after Macrolane injection for breast augmentation has been reported to be safe, and in patients treated with Macrolane, regular examination of mammography with an MRI did not appear to be necessary. The procedure can be carried out in a clean environment, keeping hygienic conditions as those required for minor surgery.

The procedure takes between thirty and ninety minutes depending on the site and quantity of gel injected. After a treatment with Macrolane, the results can be seen instantly. Some common injection-related reactions might occur including redness, swelling, tenderness, pain, bruising, or itching. Reactions normally resolve spontaneously within a few weeks. During the first week after the treatment the client should avoid strenuous exercise or any activity that could put pressure on the treatment area. It is strongly recommended to avoid exposing the treated area to intense heat or cold.

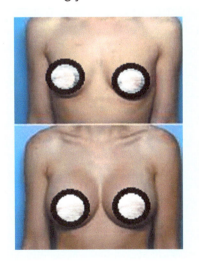

Figure 10.9. Breast augmentation by Macrolane

Macrolane can be used for breast shaping in women whom have asymmetry, loss of volume as a result of breast feeding or weight loss, or underdeveloped breasts. It is suitable for women for increasing breast size by a cup size without the need for surgery. Lower image is after the procedure.

BIO-ALCAMID

Bio-Alcamid is a stable nontoxic dermal filler that is compatible with the body. Bio-Alcamid is principally used for severe facial volume loss frequently seen as a result of antiviral drugs taken in the treatment of HIV. Severe facial volume loss due to aging, trauma, and disease can be treated with large-volume injectable fillers such as Bio-Alcamid. It is injected in the subcutaneous facial area where the volume is lost. Because these fillers should be injected with a large-bore needle, they are considered a surgically injectable insert. Large-volume dermal filler injections require anesthesia administration. Candidates for Bio-Alcamid injection require orally taken prophylactic antibiotics, starting the day before the procedure and continuing for five days. Complications may include infection, but it is very uncommon. Partial removal of the implant may be necessary to help the infection resolve if infection occurs.

SILICONE OIL

Silicon 1000 is permanent dermal filler made up of silicone oil and is commonly used to eliminate scarring from acne, or any smaller indentations of the face or body, and lip enhancement. Microdroplet silicone oil or liquid injectable silicone is also used to treat HIV-related facial lipoatrophy. Injections of silicone oil are not approved for cosmetic use in the United States. SilSkin, a purified silicone oil used for facial augmentation, has not been approved by the FDA for any medical use or for any cosmetic purpose, including the treatment of facial defects or wrinkles or enlarging the breasts.

The adverse effects of liquid silicone injections have included movement of the silicone to other parts of the body, inflammation and discoloration of surrounding tissues, and the formation of granulomas. The injection of silicone oil may trigger a foreign body response in which the foreign object is either broken down or engulfed and moved to other organs for excretion. Silicone oil cannot be broken down by the body. As the result, lower molecular silicones are removed, but the higher viscosities remain behind and are encapsulated. The body forms collagen layers around the silicone and, eventually augmentation occurs, in the form of fibrous tissue. Excess collagen formation may occur around the product, eventually causing a firm nodule. Therefore, augmentation is not due to the product itself, and large amounts of silicone oil should not be injected for volume augmentation.

FIBRIN-PLATELET FILL (SELPHYL)

A fibrin-platelet fill is a safe and rapid preparation of an activated platelet-rich fibrin matrix (PRFM) known by its trade name Selphyl. This procedure of nonsurgical cosmetics involves the collection of a small volume of the client's blood and the separation and concentration of platelets and fibrin with centrifugation force. The resulting product is treated as dermal filler for its own donor and can be injected in the face or body, where is aimed at skin rejuvenation.

Hence, the patient's own platelets naturally fill skin depressions, acne scars, wrinkles, and folds rather than using synthetic, plastic, or animal-derived materials. This preparation method of fibrin and platelets is free of red or white blood cells and provides live and intact platelets. Platelets release cytokines and growth factors, particularly platelet-derived growth factor and transforming growth factor-beta, which promote cell migration, proliferation, differentiation, and tissue growth. Transforming growth factor-beta specifically stimulates deep dermal fibroblasts to synthesize more collagen at the site of injection. The system is a novel and simple and has minimal or no allergic reaction.

PLATELET-RICH PLASMA THERAPY

Many cytokines and growth factors are implicated in the wound repair and tissue regeneration. The prospective benefits of enhanced healing processes for collagen depletion, skin depressions, wrinkles, and acne scars have led to the interest in the use of PRP (platelet rich plasma) therapy for cosmetic enhancement. Although clinicians have used PRP therapy since the mid-1990s to aid bone healing after spinal injury and soft tissue recovery following plastic surgery, it has only been in the recent years that the treatment for aesthetic purposes has come to the front position.

The appeal of PRP is that it may abundantly provide healing factors in the body's physiological conditions. Since platelets are involved in healing and hemostasis, as well as in providing growth factors to stimulate tissue regeneration and repair, it possesses the potential to stimulate collagen genesis. PRP may affect tissue healing via growth factors that are released after platelet degranulation. An injection of a concentrated version of PRP (hcPRP) is utilized for the treatment of fine lines, wrinkles, folds, and collagen loss. Although hcPRP can be injected into the same areas as common cosmetic fillers, it cannot compensate for major volume loss.

Before the treatment, the client's own blood will be taken and platelet-rich plasma will be separated from the other blood components. Then the concentrated platelets in the area targeted for the treatment will be injected. The growth factors that the platelets secrete may promote tissue regeneration and the growth of collagen. Transforming growth factor–beta is the major cytokine involved in collagen synthesis. The autologous nature of the treatment of PRP (using the patient's own blood) eliminates the risk of immune rejection or disease transmission. Depending on the degree and extent of the wrinkles or folds, typically one to three treatment sessions are required. Injections are usually spaced four to six weeks apart. The area may feel slightly warm and inflamed. Minimal discomfort may persist for few days. However, the regenerative repair process takes weeks to months.

Figure 10.10

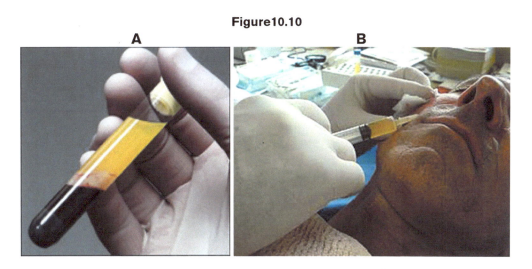

A small volume of the patient's blood is collected, and the platelets and fibrin are concentrated during a simple centrifuge process (A). The resulting product (liquid, gel or membrane) can be applied to a treatment area of the face or body to stimulate natural new tissue growth (B).

DERMAL FILLER INJECTION TECHNIQUES

Before injection, the skin must be cleansed and disinfected. Depending on the length and extent of the procedure, local anesthesia may be applied with a small-bore (30- or 32-gauge) needle. Local anesthesia can be used in conjugation with ice packs, numbing cream, or dental freezing. Physicians may choose to numb or anaesthetize the treatment area to further minimize discomfort. The cosmetic filler should be carefully implanted under the skin where it is needed, and the smoothness of the tissues must be ensured by gentle massaging of the treated area. Filler is injected directly into the skin using a fine needle (27 G × 1/2 in. size) to reduce injection discomfort. At the conclusion of the treatment, the skin must be cleansed thoroughly. Makeup can be applied after the procedure if desired. The follow-up appointment can be scheduled in one to two weeks if needed.

There are five recognized techniques used for injecting dermal fillers:

1. *The linear retrotracing or linear threading techniques:* this method is used for filling fine or superficial wrinkles. The needle inserted in the dermis with a fifteen-degree angle, and the dermal filler is injected in a linear pattern while withdrawing or retreating the syringe in the same line without applying pressure.
2. *The sandwich technique:* it is a preferred method to treat, in a same area, a facial depression or fold and fine wrinkles. Multiple lines may be injected parallel to each other at the same area.
3. *The fan technique:* this method is adapted for enhancing tissue volume in areas such as the nasolabial triangle. Multiple injections are performed in different directions without exiting the needle tip from the surface of skin. The fan technique allows for covering of a large area while minimizing the number of needle puncture sites.
4. *The serial puncture technique:* this technique consists of a linear series of small quantities of filler that is injected along the same wrinkle sufficiently close together to avoid any irregularity or empty space.
5. *The crosshatching technique:* this method is suitable for modifying facial contours and enhancing tissue volume. It consists of a series of injections using the linear threading techniques that are parallel to each other, with the next series of perpendicular injections pattern in same layer of the skin.

Figure 10.11: Dermal filler injection methods

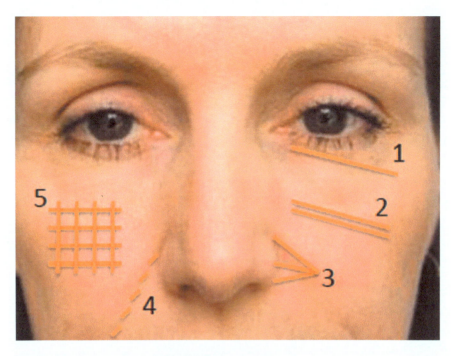

1- **Linear threading**
2- **Sandwich**
3- **Fan**
4- **Serial puncture**
5- **Cross Hatching**

TYPICAL SITES OF INJECTIONS

In general, injectable products are used in the lower two-thirds of the face, mainly for lip enhancement, wrinkles, and folds around the lips and nose. They can also be used for correcting folds and wrinkles on the forehead and also for the crow's feet. Using injectable fillers, the cosmetic physician can remodel the cheekbones, soften facial contours, fill in wrinkles and lines, increase and remodel lips, and straighten the nose bumps to enhance its shape and appearance. However, cosmetic filler injection is a state of the art procedure, and the cosmetic physician makes judgments as the best choice of treatment at the time of assessment.

Figure 10.12 illustrates typical injection sites for the dermal fillers. Initial treatment sessions involve a consultation with the cosmetic physician, who will review the client's medical history, discuss the history of previous use of fillers or other cosmetic procedures, check whether there are any contraindications for using a filler (including pregnancy, breastfeeding, allergy to any component of the filler, and skin infection). The physician should also review the client's cosmetic needs and expectations and suggest which filler is the most appropriate to use. Below the most common areas of dermal filler treatment are summarized and illustrated:

- horizontal forehead lines
- vertical lines between the brows
- nasolabial folds (beside nose)
- marionette lines (beside mouth)
- lip wrinkling, volume, and size
- depressed scars
- lip, cheek, and prejowl groove
- frown lines
- eyebrows
- cheeks/midface
- ear lobes
- angle of jaw
- nose
- chin
- crow's feet
- temples

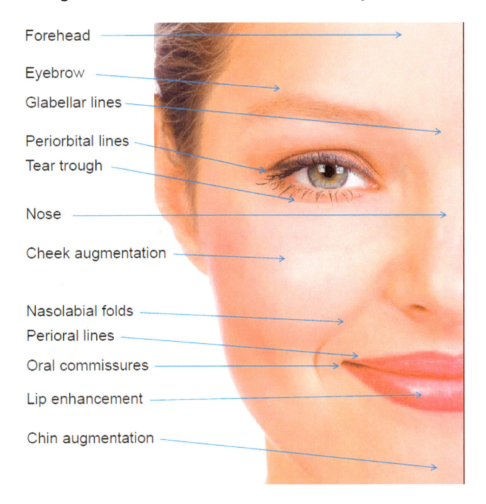

Figure 10.12. Most common dermal filler injection sites

Dermal fillers can be used to correct problem areas such as laugh lines, smile lines, smoker's lines, and marionette lines, but there are also ways to use dermal fillers to enhance certain features. The most popular being the cheekbones, chins, jawlines and eyebrows. Treatment can take as short a time as thirty minutes, depending on the number of injection sites and the injectables used. These injections are virtually painless, and the results can be seen almost immediately.

NONSURGICAL RHINOPLASTY (NOSE JOB)

Having a decent nose shape is a desire of almost everyone. The nose is the first facial feature that get noticed, simply because it is in the middle of the face and is always exposed. Therefore, people turn to rhinoplasty not only to change their nose but also the appearance of their entire face. That is the reason for high demand of rhinoplasty as compared to other cosmetic surgery corrections. Rhinoplasty is also commonly called "nose reshaping" or a "nose job."

The most common motivation for having a nose job is imperfections, such as a hump on the bridge, a concave nose bridge, a droopy tip, or a short nose bridge. Traditional surgical nose jobs can be quite costly and painful, with long recovery times often associated with postsurgery bruising and bleeding. Patients who are interested in nose surgery may be astonished to discover a nonsurgical procedure, which is an excellent alternative to the traditional surgically invasive rhinoplasty. Interestingly, a nonsurgical nose reshaping involves using injectable hyaluronic acid gels such as Restylane, Teosyal, Juvederm, or Calcium Hydroxylapatite Radiesse to shape and contour the nose.

Distinct from surgical practice, these fillers allow candidates to achieve fast results with no or little healing time. Therefore, nonsurgical nose jobs using dermal fillers is a practical and realistic alternative, which allows clients to see a desired outcome in the appearance of their nose and face in general in a timely and costly manner. Practically, a hump can be minimized by adding long-lasting fillers to the front nasal angle. Botox can also be used to lift the tip of the nose, which may have drooped because of the aging process. Results can last for months or years, delaying or in some cases eliminating the need for traditional surgery.

When nasal imbalance is inconsiderable, a nonsurgical nose reshaping can offer patients with exceptional results and an improved overall appearance. Unfortunately, those with considerable nasal imperfections and those who are looking to reduce the size of their nose are not candidates for the nonsurgical nose reshaping procedure.

Figure 10.12 Nonsurgical nose job

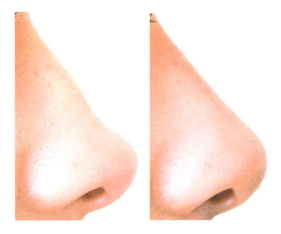

With the sense of a true cosmetic surgery artist, noses can be aesthetically reshaped to the desired form. Holes can be filled in, bumps made to disappear and can be smoothed out by building up the surrounding low areas, tips can be elevated, and scars can be filled in. A nose that may first appear to require a surgical correction may in fact be simply improved with dermal filler injection.

INJECTABLES: RISKS AND SIDE EFFECTS

The risks associated with injectable fillers involve bruising and some temporary swelling or infection. With the use of dental freezing, the treated area may be somewhat swollen for two hours postoperation. Swellings due to implants can resolve in one to two days. There is risk of developing transient facial redness over the implant, but it usually resolves very quickly. There is also a risk of bruising that normally disappears in few days, but it can readily be concealed with a makeup. Using fillers usually does not require any allergy skin tests.

There can be some side effects, mainly related to the injection as opposed to the product itself, such as swelling, pain, itching, discoloration, tenderness, and sometimes redness. Typically, these disappear within a day or two after the injection in skin and within a week after injection to the lips. Possible side effects are mild to moderate in nature and relatively short lasting.

These side effects may include temporary skin reactions such as redness, tenderness, and bruising, which are easily covered with light makeup. If bruising is a concern, it is recommended that seven days prior to the appointment the client avoid aspirin that thins the blood and vitamin E that can result in more bruising. The clients must avoid ibuprofen (Advil, Motrin) and anti-inflammatory drugs (Aleve, naproxen) for three days prior to the appointment.

Taking Tylenol (acetaminophen) is not a concern for the development of bruising. Some suggest avoiding herbal medications such as ginkgo biloba for three days prior to undergoing the procedure. A possible delayed side effect can be small bumps under the skin. These bumps may not be visible and can be noticed only when one presses on the area. The bumps usually go away on their own, although occasionally visible bumps have been reported.

DERMAL FILLER PREOPERATIONAL CHECKLIST

Nonsurgical medical aesthetic procedures such as peels and laser treatments may be performed by nonphysicians in a spa setting. Nonsurgical procedures, although not invasive, carry some risk and should be researched carefully. Medical aesthetics practitioners should be prepared to answer common questions that their clients may ask before going through the procedure. The following are some important points to consider and inquire about prior to consenting to a nonsurgical procedure:

1. What risks are associated with the procedure?
2. How is the treatment administered?
3. Is the procedure painful, and if so, what sort of pain relief is available?
4. How long does the procedure take?
5. Is the equipment sterile?
6. Will there be any temporary side effects?

7. What symptoms might be considered serious where urgent care is required?
8. How long do the results last?
9. Is the facility licensed?
10. Who will be administering the treatment?
11. What qualifications, training, and experience does he/she have?
12. Does the treatment require the supervision of a physician?
13. Are the staff willing to discuss the price for the procedures?

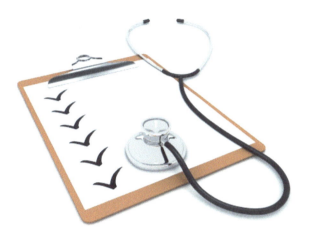

Lightning Source UK Ltd.
Milton Keynes UK
UKHW050001160519
342754UK00004B/41/P